THE
SKINNY
ON FAT

OTHER BOOKS BY M. SARA ROSENTHAL

The Gastrointestinal Sourcebook (1997, 1998)
The Breastfeeding Sourcebook (2nd edition, 1998)
The Breast Sourcebook (2nd edition, 1999)
The Pregnancy Sourcebook (3rd edition, 1999)
The Thyroid Sourcebook for Women (1999)
The Type 2 Diabetic Woman (1999)
The Thyroid Sourcebook (4th edition, 2000)
Women and Depression (2000)
Women and Passion (Canada only, 2000)
Women of the '60s Turning 50 (Canada only, 2000)
Managing PMS Naturally (2001)
The Canadian Type 2 Diabetes Sourcebook (Canada only, 2002)
The Fertility Sourcebook (3rd edition, 2002)
The Hypothyroid Sourcebook (2002)
*The Natural Woman's Guide to
Preventing Diabetes Complications* (2002)
Women Managing Stress (2002)
The Gynecological Sourcebook (4th edition, 2003)
[Canadian edition of above: *Gynecological Health*]
*The Natural Woman's Guide to
Hormone Replacement Therapy* (2003)

50 WAYS SERIES
50 Ways to Prevent Colon Cancer (2000)
50 Ways Women Can Prevent Heart Disease (2000)
50 Ways to Manage Type 2 Diabetes (U.S. only, 2001)
50 Ways to Manage Ulcer, Heartburn and Reflux (2001)
50 Ways to Prevent and Manage Stress (2001)
50 Ways to Prevent Depression Without Drugs (2001)

THE
SKINNY
ON FAT

A Look at Low-Fat Culture

M. SARA ROSENTHAL, Ph.D.

M&S

National Library of Canada Cataloguing in Publication

Rosenthal, M. Sara
The skinny on fat : a look at low-fat culture / M. Sara Rosenthal.

Includes bibliographical references and index.
ISBN 0-7710-7573-1

1. Nutrition–Popular works. 2. Obesity–Health aspects. 3. Weight loss–Health aspects. 4. Reducing diets–Health aspects. 5. Body image. I. Title.

RC628.R68 2004   613.2   C2003-905819-0

We acknowledge the financial support of the Government of Canada through the Book Publishing Industry Development Program and that of the Government of Ontario through the Ontario Media Development Corporation's Ontario Book Initiative. We further acknowledge the support of the Canada Council for the Arts and the Ontario Arts Council for our publishing program.

Typeset in Sabon by M&S, Toronto
Printed and bound in Canada

This book is printed on acid-free paper that is
100% ancient forest friendly (100% post-consumer recycled).

McClelland & Stewart Ltd.
The Canadian Publishers
481 University Avenue
Toronto, Ontario
M5G 2E9
www.mcclelland.com

1   2   3   4   5   08   07   06   05   04

IMPORTANT NOTICE

The purpose of this book is to educate. It is sold with the understanding that the author and publisher shall have neither liability nor responsibility for any injury caused or alleged to be caused directly or indirectly by the information contained in this book. While every effort has been made to ensure its accuracy, the book's contents should not be construed as medical advice. Each person's health needs are unique. To obtain recommendations appropriate to your particular situation, please consult a qualified health-care provider. The herbal information in this book is provided for education purposes only and is not meant to be used without consulting a qualified health practitioner who is trained in herbal medicine.

Not all source materials are cited within the text. Please consult the Bibliography for a complete list of resources.

All dollar values are in U.S. dollars unless otherwise noted.

SARAHEALTHGUIDES™

These are M. Sara Rosenthal's own line of health books written by her and by other health authors. SarahealthGuides are dedicated to rare, controversial, or stigmatizing health topics you won't find in regular bookstores. SarahealthGuides are available at on-line bookstores or toll-free at 1-866-752-6820. Visit <www.sarahealth.com> for upcoming titles.

Contents

ACKNOWLEDGMENTS

I wish to thank the following people (listed alphabetically), whose expertise and dedication helped to lay so much of the groundwork for this book: Gillian Arsenault, M.D., CC.F.P., IB.L.C., F.R.C.P.; Pamela Craig, M.D., F.A.C.S., Ph.D.; Masood Kahthamee, M.D., F.A.C.O.G.; Debra Lander, M.D., F.R.C.P.; Gary May, M.D., F.R.C.P.; James McSherry, M.B., Ch.B., F.C.F.P., FR.C.G.P., F.A.A.F.P., F.A.B.M.P.; Suzanne Pratt, M.D., FA.C.OG.; Wm Warren Rudd, M.D., F.R.C.S., F.A.C.S., colon and rectal surgeon and founder and director of the Rudd Clinic for Diseases of the Colon and Rectum (Toronto); and Robert Volpe, M.D., F.R.C.P., F.A.C.P.

William Harvey, Ph.D., L.L.B., University of Toronto Joint Centre for Bioethics, whose devotion to bioethics has inspired me, continues to support my work and makes it possible for me to have the courage to question and challenge issues in health care and medical ethics. Irving Rootman, Ph.D., former director, University of Toronto Centre for Health Promotion, continues to encourage my interest in primary prevention and health promotion issues. Helen Lenskyj, Ph.D., professor, Department of Sociology and Equity Studies, Ontario Institute for Studies in Education/University of Toronto, and Laura M. Purdy, Ph.D., philosopher and bioethicist, Wells College, Ithaca, N.Y., have been central figures in my understanding the complexities of feminist bioethics. Meredith Schwartz, my editorial and research assistant, worked very hard to make this book come into being. And finally, thanks to Patricia Kennedy, my editor at McClelland & Stewart Ltd., who championed this project.

I'm also grateful to my husband, Kenneth B. Ain, M.D., who gave me valuable insights into diet and nutrition from his perspective as an endocrinologist.

INTRODUCTION

Remember the old nursery rhyme: "Jack Sprat could eat no fat, His wife could eat no lean, And so betwixt them both, They licked the platter clean." We in North America are so saturated with fat and diet information – conflicting studies and nutrition guidelines have made us so confused – that we don't know how to eat anymore. We are living the nursery rhyme. These days, it's not unusual to find a Sprat couple on different, if not opposing, diets. One may be on the Ornish-style very low-fat diet, which limits daily calorie intake from fat to 10 per cent; the other may be on an Atkins-style diet, which limits daily calorie intake from carbohydrates to less than 10 per cent. And in both cases, the diets may fail to produce any results.

Then we're told that there are good fats and bad fats, good cholesterol and bad cholesterol, good carbohydrates and bad carbohydrates. We're so inundated with information on dietary components, we're afraid to shop for food anymore.

We are obsessed as a culture with low fat and weight loss, yet statistics show we're getting fatter, and obesity-related conditions, such as cardiovascular disease and type 2 diabetes, are on the rise.

I recently read that theaters in London built in the 1800s are losing money, because North American tourists can no longer fit in the narrow seats; the English are having to retrofit their buildings to accommodate our fat.

As convenience food and fast-food eating have become the norm, and as we have practically engineered physical activity out of our lives (particularly in car-dominated suburbia), we are seeing the consequences in our children. Never before has childhood obesity in North America been so high. Children are being diagnosed in record numbers with high cholesterol, type 2 diabetes, and other conditions normally not seen until adulthood. Our children are the least fit generation of children; they are suffering from malnutrition in the form of *overnutrition*.

And although obesity is on the rise, media images of "thinness" pervade, creating a fear of fat, or fat phobia, that is also out of control. Many people who are not medically obese (as defined in Chapter 1) still perceive themselves to be overweight or obese and will pursue a diet unnecessarily. This frequently leads to catastrophic eating behaviors and disorders.

It is my hope that this book will give you some insights into why we are ballooning, and will help you to think critically and to question the health claims surrounding diets, weight-loss products, and medical-journal studies you see quoted in the news. I've tried to give you the book I needed and wanted about diet and fat that I couldn't seem to find for myself.

When it comes to the subject of diet, "fat," and body image, I wear several hats. As author of more than twenty-five consumer health books, I have been immersed in diet and nutrition information for more than a decade, and still find the published studies confusing, if not contradictory. For example, there are many "fat acceptance" movements and critics of obesity research, which point out that being overweight is not necessarily an unhealthy state. They claim that the studies quoting deaths linked to obesity are inaccurate and only serve to promote the multibillion-dollar weight-loss and diet industry. But as someone who has written several books about obesity-related conditions, such as type 2 diabetes, I know that the studies that point to obesity as a cause of morbidity and death refer to the complications of obesity: the obesity-related diseases that develop due to strain on the body. While there are those who can be fat and fit, and maintain lifelong health and wellness, *being fat and unfit* – the state, sadly, most people who are struggling with obesity are in – is indeed an unhealthy state that breeds chronic illnesses such as cardiovascular disease and type 2 diabetes. In most people, obesity will naturally occur when our energy intake is greater than our energy output. In short, when we eat more calories than we're burning up in activity, most of us are genetically wired and biologically engineered to get fat.

As a medical sociologist, I am also questioning how our society has contributed to changes in our diet and our perceptions of weight. For example, our bodies have never before lived in a time where food was so available or abundant. To our ancient biology, which hasn't changed in thousands of years, *this is pretty new*. We survived and evolved by protecting ourselves from weight loss and storing calories as fat.

As a bioethicist (a.k.a. medical ethicist), I am looking at ethical problems with diet claims, misinformation about weight gain and weight loss that may prove harmful to the consumer, as well as whether nutrition labels and label claims may be misleading – either overpromising or not disclosing pertinent information to the consumer.

Finally, as any researcher, I must also locate myself within this book: I am a woman who has turned forty, who is bombarded with the same media images of youth, beauty, and thinness as any other woman. At the same time, I notice real changes in my metabolism, and the need to increase my physical activity and decrease my calorie intake. Given the demands on my time, and my love of culinary pleasures, I have the same struggles and challenges in staying healthy as all of you. Because of gender differences in body image and social position, women are the lead consumers of weight-loss products and information. The number of overweight women will increase by 12 per cent by 2005. It's estimated that $92.7 million in sales of these products and services are due to women trying to lose weight for health reasons. Appearance-driven women dieters will add another $68 million in sales. The Food Marketing Institute in Washington, D.C., and Atlanta's Calorie Control Council confirmed that nearly nine in ten women used low-fat foods and 85 per cent used low-calorie products last year.

I also look at these issues through a parental lens; I have several close friends whose children are obese due to many of the cultural shifts I point out in this book. Thus I have tried to create a book that gives you the skinny on all things fat. Ultimately, our current obesity epidemic on the one hand and eating disorder epidemic on the other exist within a socio-economic and political context, and we should all be aware of this. For example, the food industry and the food lobby influence our eating habits and purchases. With all the confusing labeling and low-fat misinformation, it's easy to get fatter on low-fat products than you think, as this book explains.

This book also explains the confusion – and hidden agendas – behind the studies and the health claims: the heart-health and diet studies, the wine studies, the olive-oil studies, and the studies comparing various diets to each other are all examined.

This book also takes a good look at dietary fat and cancer, anti-obesity drugs, over-the-counter weight-loss products, and nutriceuticals such as fat replacers and sweeteners.

By the time you finish *The Skinny on Fat*, you'll appreciate the complexities of "fat" and understand how in most instances "getting fat" and "getting thin" are multifactorial processes that have much more to do with our eating behaviors, evolutionary biology, nutrition literacy, genetics, gender, and our particularly fortunate economic and social location in this world than you might think.

CHAPTER 1

WHY WE ARE GETTING FATTER:

The Obesity Issue

At the eighty-fifth annual meeting of the Endocrine Society in Philadelphia in 2003, the latest obesity research was presented, which concluded that the North American lifestyle was the single, largest contributing factor to obesity. Although social, behavioral, metabolic, cellular, and molecular factors all contribute to obesity, obesity genes were found to be "turned on" only when they were exposed to an environment conducive to weight gain, such as the North American environment.

North Americans have the highest obesity rates in the world. More than half of North American adults and about 25 per cent of North American children are now obese. These figures reflect a doubling of the adult obesity rate since the 1960s, and a doubling of the childhood obesity rate since the late 1970s – a staggering increase when you think about it in raw numbers. Obese children will most likely grow up to become obese adults, according to the most recent research.

The U.S. Centers for Disease Control (CDC) has tracked obesity rates by state, considering gender, age, race, and education level. In 1991, only four states had obesity rates of 15 per cent or higher; today, at least thirty-seven states do. The CDC study compared the spread of obesity throughout the United States to the spread of a communicable disease during an epidemic. In Canada, the rates of obesity are climbing at an equal speed, particularly in our aboriginal communities and non-white populations. Obesity is now second only to smoking as a leading cause of death. In the United States alone, obesity-related health-care costs are close to $240 billion. In Canada, the costs are projected to topple our health-care system. One in four Canadians older than forty-five, for example, now has type 2 diabetes, a classic obesity-related chronic disease.

For many years, people have been hearing that obesity is caused by sedentary living and by eating too much of the wrong foods. In other words, obesity is caused by an energy imbalance: consuming more calories than can be burned off through regular activity. That's still true, but now researchers who look at nutrition through a socio-political and ethical lens are beginning to hold the food industry more accountable for the obesity increase through its advertising, spending, and lobbying practices, as well as questionable influences on schools and nutritional researchers. All of this is corrupting the way our children live and eat, and the way nutrition labeling and guidelines are developed. As adult consumers, we have become confused by what we see on food labels and in printed guidelines. Even when those of us who are not suffering from disordered eating (see Chapter 2) consciously try to select what we think are more nutritious foods, we still frequently wind up consuming hidden calories.

Other changes in our society have contributed to obesity too. We are more sedentary due to long commutes, bigger and better televisions, digital cable, "strip mall" living that makes it harder to do errands on foot (endemic in the suburbs), as well as the rise of the computer and the Internet. Our children are no longer encouraged to walk to school or to play outside in many neighborhoods because of safety considerations. Many parents are opting for safer indoor activities, fearing their children will be hurt or will vanish. In many communities, budget cuts have led schools to eliminate their physical-education programs and facilities. In urban communities, there are fewer green spaces and parks, which are replaced by malls (always with food courts) and parking lots. People are working harder to make the same wages, and two-income families are more stretched and stressed each year. Alongside these changes, the fast-food industry has experienced enormous growth, making more high-fat, inexpensive meals widely available. Thus convenience food, as it is also called, has become the standard North American diet. This chapter outlines the socio-economic causes of obesity, which are more complex than you might assume.

DEFINING OBESITY

Obesity refers to a body size that is too fat for good health. Obese people have greater incidences of heart attacks, strokes, peripheral vascular disease (circulation problems, leading to many other health problems), type 2 diabetes, and certain types of cancers (see Chapter 3). Obesity is also a culturally unacceptable body size, which can lead to problems with self-esteem (see Chapter 2).

At one time, anyone who weighed 20 per cent more than their ideal weight for their age and height was defined as clinically "obese." But this is not as accurate an indicator as the Body Mass Index (BMI), which is now the best measurement of obesity. The BMI is calculated by dividing your weight (in kilograms) by your height (in meters) squared. (The formula used is BMI=kg÷m² if you're doing this on your calculator.) BMI charts can be found on the backs of cereal boxes, in numerous health magazines, and, of course, on the Internet, where you simply type in your weight in pounds and your height in inches to arrive at your BMI. As of this writing, a good BMI calculator can be found at <www.consumer.gov/weightloss/bmi.htm>. (Or type in the key words *BMI Chart* on your search engine.)

Currently on the Web site I refer to, a BMI of 18.5 or less indicates that you are underweight. A BMI between 18.5 and 24.9 is normal. The most recent clinical guidelines define people with a BMI between 25 and 29.9 as overweight, and those with a BMI between 30 and 34.9 as obese (mild to moderate). A BMI between 35.0 and 39.9 would indicate the severely obese; people with a BMI of 40 or greater are considered morbidly obese. These BMI guidelines to calculate obesity match the clinical guidelines for defining obesity as of 1998. Since the guidelines have changed, roughly 72 million more North Americans who were not considered obese in 1998 are now considered obese. The guidelines for what constitutes type 2 diabetes similarly changed in 1998, which also means that more people who would not have been diagnosed prior to the changes have now been told they have diabetes. This has also helped the diet industry and some food lobbies to sell people on particular types of diets, leading to more confusion than ever (see Chapters 4, 5, and 7).

Obesity is not an eating disorder but can be the result of compulsive overeating, known as binge eating disorder (BED), discussed in Chapter 2. Roughly 20 to 46 per cent of obese people suffer from BED.

Obesity rates in children and teens are calculated through BMIs that are at or above sex- and age-specific weights within the ninety-fifty percentiles. This is a more conservative approach to account for growing spurts.

PHYSIOLOGICAL CAUSES OF OBESITY

The main physiological cause of obesity, to repeat, is eating more calories than you burn. People gain weight for two reasons: they may eat excessively (often excessive amounts of nutritious foods), which results in daily consumption of too many calories; or they may eat moderately but simply be too inactive for the calories they *do* ingest. Genetic makeup can predispose some body types to obesity earlier in life because of "thrifty genes" (see below). But in general, experts in nutrition agree that genetics plays only a *small* role in the sharp increase in obesity seen in the last thirty years. Since genetic changes take place over centuries, and our obesity rate has at least doubled since the 1960s, it's fairly obvious that lifestyle factors are the chief culprit. Studies and surveys show that we are actually eating about 500 calories more than we were in the 1970s; we're up from 3,300 calories per day (per person) to 3,800 per day per person. Frequent snacking, encouraged by the food industry's development and marketing of more innovative and tempting snacks, has been cited as one of the most apparent changes in our eating patterns during the last thirty years. In fact, it is worse than that. The practice of snacking has doubled from the mid-1980s to the mid-1990s. The fast-food invasion, of course, has also contributed to the increase.

THRIFTY GENES

Genetics plays a role in obesity when it comes to aboriginal and other minority groups, due to what some researchers call the "thrifty gene." This is the gene thought to be responsible for the higher rates of obesity and obesity-related conditions in aboriginal and non-European populations. This means that the more recently your culture has lived indigenously or nomadically (living off the land you came from and eating seasonally or indigenously), the more efficient your metabolism is. Unfortunately, it is also more sensitive to *nutrient excess*. If you're an aboriginal North American, only about one hundred years have passed since your ancestors lived indigenously. This is an exceedingly short amount of time to ask thousands of years of hunter-gatherer genes to adjust to the terrible convenience-food diet prevalent in North America. If you're of African descent, you haven't lived here any longer than about four hundred years; prior to that, your ancestors were living a tribal, nomadic lifestyle. Again, four hundred years is *not* a long time.

As for Hispanic populations or other immigrant populations, many come from families who have spent generations in poverty.

Their metabolisms adjusted to long periods of famine, and are often overloaded by our abundance of high-caloric foods.

Asian populations generally have the lowest rates of obesity, but that is because they are frequently able to maintain their dietary habits when they emigrate to North America. In fact, European North Americans tend to benefit when they adopt the same diets. That said, when Asian and Southeast Asian populations begin eating the North American way – pizzas, hamburgers, fries, sweet drinks, and snack foods – their obesity rates begin to soar too, and they are more prone to type 2 diabetes.

Thrifty genes are evident when you look at the obesity patterns in the United States. There, obesity is more prevalent in African Americans, Latinos, Native Americans, and Native Hawaiians and American Samoans; these groups have a higher incidence of diabetes and cardiovascular disease as well. For example, almost 63 per cent of Native Hawaiian women are obese, and between 61 and 75 per cent of Yaqui Indians are overweight. Among Hispanics, Mexicans have the highest rates of obesity (48.2 per cent), followed by Puerto Ricans (40.2 per cent).

Cultural attitudes about body image may also play a role in the disparity between obesity rates among non-European North Americans. Black women (both Caribbean and African American) are not as susceptible to images of thinness as white women, and do not feel the same cultural pressures to be thin. That's because a fuller figure is considered more attractive by their culture, unlike the case in white culture. The fear of obesity, which inversely contributes to it among women who do "prophylactic dieting" (see Chapter 2), is not as much of a factor in non-Europeans.

Diets of poverty may also be a factor, particularly on reserves in Canada, where food availability in northern stores is a problem. Diets of poverty – wherever they're found – typically rely on calories from high-fat, low-nutrient foods instead of fresher foods, fruits, and vegetables. Aboriginal, African, and Hispanic populations tend to have much lower incomes, and are therefore eating lower-quality food, which, when combined with the "thrifty gene," can lead to obesity and obesity-related health problems. When epidemiologists look at these same "thrifty gene" groups in people of higher-income levels who can afford healthier foods, the obesity rates are lower.

MORBID OBESITY

Morbid obesity is extreme obesity. People with BMIs in the high 30s or over 40 are classified as morbidly obese. Another method for calculating morbid obesity is by ideal body weight: when people exceed their ideal weight by more than one hundred pounds, they are considered morbidly obese. People who are morbidly obese are at the highest risk of health complications. Morbidly obese men aged between twenty-five and thirty-five have twelve times the risk of dying prematurely than their peers of normal weights. Morbid obesity also causes a range of medical problems, such as breathing difficulties, gastrointestinal ailments, endocrine problems (especially diabetes), musculoskeletal problems, hygiene problems, sexual problems, and so on. Some people are now forced to undergo bariatric surgery (the stomach-stapling procedure) in order to lower their risk of dying from their fat. It's important to clarify that surgery for morbid obesity is not plastic surgery; it is serious gastrointestinal surgery that carries significant risks, offered only to those people whose weight poses an immediate health risk and who have not been able to find any other way to lose weight. For more information, visit the Association for Morbid Obesity Support at <www.obesityhelp.com/morbidobesity>.

SIZING UP OUR CHILDREN

In the 2001 film *Monster's Ball* (for which Halle Berry won the Best Actress Oscar), a poor African-American waitress (Berry) struggles to raise her son alone, and later comes to grips with his accidental death. Her son, who we presume is under twelve, is morbidly obese, which clearly enrages her. As she steps out to run an errand, he quickly sneaks a candy bar into his mouth, cramming it in as though he were starving. When Berry returns and catches him in the act, she hits him and calls him "fatty" in an ineffective discipline tantrum. The boy goes into his room, crying, withdraws more candy from his stash, and, once again, eats to comfort himself. This horribly pathetic scene, although an extreme example of childhood obesity, touched the hearts of millions of parents who can relate in some way.

Despite their nutritional knowledge or economic circumstances, however, many parents of mild, moderate, or severely obese children are often frustrated in their efforts to stop their children from getting fatter. It is a battle they are losing, thanks to the infiltration of corporate greed into our children's minds and schools. Canadian health-care practitioners bemoan the rise of type 2 diabetes in aboriginal children, a trend now starting to be seen in children of other cultures.

Children today spend about twenty-two hours per week in front of the television, consuming high-fat snacks while watching advertisements for more high-fat snacks. If you count computer time, videos, and video games, many children spend thirty-eight hours a week in front of some type of screen, which almost equals the hours spent on the average full-time job. Children watch more than thirty thousand commercials per year, and roughly 25 per cent of North American children between the ages of two and five actually have a TV in their bedrooms.

In addition, since improving a child's diet often means altering the whole family's eating patterns, changing poor dietary habits is difficult. Many children come from families with terrible eating patterns: they skip breakfast, snack all day, and have huge dinners with desserts. This diet paves the way to childhood obesity.

A recent study in the *Canadian Medical Association Journal* found that almost 30 per cent of boys and 24 per cent of girls aged seven to thirteen were overweight in 1996. Only 15 per cent of each group had been overweight fifteen years earlier.

CREATING OBESITY THROUGH ADVERTISING

There is a direct connection between obesity and television commercials. Several studies have documented that children who watch television (commercials included) are fatter than those who don't.

Since the 1980s, we have seen a virtual explosion in advertising to children, mostly to promote food. In 1987, researchers who surveyed advertising on Saturday-morning network television counted 225 advertisements; 71 per cent were junk-food ads. The number of commercials increased to 997 in 1994; the majority of the ads, again, were for junk foods: sweet cereal, candy, fast food, soft drinks, cookies, and salty snacks. Only about 2 per cent of food advertising is for "real" food, such as fruits, vegetables, grains, or beans. Regardless of whether fast or real food is advertised, 95 per cent of all food advertised to children in North America are foods high in sugar, salt, and fat.

Children are exerting pressure on their parents to purchase the goods they see. Working parents, out of guilt, feel obliged to purchase the foods that are making their children fat. Food advertisers spend an immense amount of time and energy appealing to children; for example, the most popular ads among children in surveys revealed the Taco Bell commercials featuring a talking chihuahua. Food companies spend more than $11 billion annually in North America on advertising in all media, and the figures for 1999 reflect that most of the advertising comes from fast-food companies: more than $627.2 million was spent by McDonald's in the United States alone, and $403.6 million was spent by Burger King.

Children's nagging for food products has actually been measured and analyzed by marketing experts. Parents respond to pleading nags (please, please, please!), persistent nags (repeating the request over and over), forceful nags (with threats attached, such as "I won't do my homework unless . . ."), demonstrative nags (tantrums, common in candy aisles at checkout counters), pity nags (the child claims s/he'll be harmed or shunned in some way if the product isn't bought); and sugar-coated nags (promises/declaration of love in return for the item). Food advertisers count on the children's market to increase their bottom lines; but our children's waistlines are what really expand. For example, most American children now get about 25 per cent of their total vegetable servings in the form of potato chips or french fries.

The problem of television and obesity is so endemic that the University of Alberta has designed a three-month program for children that teaches them about the benefits of exercise, watching less TV, and sticking to a healthier diet. According to the Children's Exercise and Nutrition Centre at McMaster University in Hamilton, Ontario, childhood obesity is considered to be at epidemic proportions. Genetic factors play only a small role in this problem. Although 40 per cent of children may have a tendency to become overweight, sedentary living and high-fat snacking have been identified as the switches that "trip" the obesity gene.

But limiting television time does not stop the sedentariness or the advertising. On top of their TV time, there are now those hours at their computers on the Internet, as well as several hours watching videos or playing video games.

The Internet is also a powerful tool used by fast-food companies to obtain marketing information about children. In the United States, a 1998 federal investigation of Web sites targeting children revealed that almost 90 per cent solicited personal information from them. Personal information from kids! Out of those Web sites, only 1 per cent required parental consent (which is still difficult to obtain ethically on the Internet). A character on McDonald's Web site, for example, encouraged kids to send Ronald McDonald an e-mail revealing their favorite menu item at McDonald's.

Many consumer and parent groups have sought to ban advertising to children under seven; children under seven frequently confuse the ads for programming, and are therefore more gullible targets.

But even if children were banned from watching television and using the Internet, they would be targets for fast-food advertising through promotional links between food and toy companies, and fast food and Hollywood. (Disneyland now has a McDonald's.)

Food companies even use education to influence children. One trend is to produce counting books for young children to promote arithmetic skills. These books require a parent to purchase brand-name candies, cookies, or sugar-sweetened cereals. The books instruct the children to "count" using their food item as "tokens" that are placed onto a space on the page; teachers and parents find them helpful. So do the food companies. The children become dependent on the brand to learn to count. These books also include value coupons to purchase more products and, of course, the brand is pictured on every page. More than 1.2 million copies of the Cheerios counting book sold between 1998 and 2000, no doubt selling more Cheerios too. Froot Loops and Oreo cookies books are other best-sellers. The Oreo cookies counting books instruct children to count to ten while the children eat their way down from ten to zero. Advertising is also done by branding dozens of non-related food items, such as apparel, which influence children as well.

We know from studies done in the late 1980s that children spend huge amounts of their own money on food items. At that time, children's spending averaged about $4.42 per week (which amounted to roughly $6 billion a year). Children also influenced family spending, which accounted for another $132 billion. In 1997, children aged seven to twelve spent $2.3 billion of their own money on snacks and beverages; teens that year spent $58 billion. Today, children of three to five years account for roughly $1.5 billion of food sales when spending their own money (allowance usually); they now influence an additional $15 billion. Children four to twelve spend $27 billion on food, and influence an additional $188 billion. In 2001, it was estimated that teens alone accounted for $136 billion in food sales. The 1999 figure for children's spending on food (which included influencing purchases) totaled $485 billion annually. Children control substantial markets for certain foods: salty snacks (25 per cent), soft drinks (30 per cent), frozen pizza (40 per cent), cold cereals (50 per cent), and canned pasta (60 per cent).

SOFT MONEY

One of the largest contributors to childhood obesity is the soft-drink industry. Soft-drink manufacturers have spent money to increase the amount of soft drinks North American children consume. They have even forged relationships with schools, providing them with logoed school supplies in exchange for exclusive rights to become the "brand" carried in the school district; in the United States, these are known as "pouring rights" contracts. Soft drinks marketed to children do not include diet soft drinks, which are marketed to adults; they are regular soft drinks that comprise carbonated water, about ten teaspoons of sugar, and flavors. A twelve-ounce can has about 160 calories, and contains levels of caffeine that can exceed 100 mg – a level equal to a cup of coffee. There is no nutritional value to soft drinks, which makes them the perfect junk food, or what the Center for Science in the Public Interest, a Washington, D.C.–based consumer rights think-tank, refers to as "liquid candy." Nutritionists advise that any other beverage would be better than a regular soft drink, including sweet juices, which at least have vitamins. Between 1985 and 1997, schools purchased 30 per cent less milk, while increasing their purchases of soft drinks by 1,100 per cent.

The greatest access to soft drinks in schools is provided through vending machines. Today, twelve-ounce cans are routinely replaced with twenty-ounce cans, encouraging children to ingest larger quantities. Convenient screw-top plastic bottles enable children to carry their drinks around all day long, sipping regularly, which has increased the number of cavities and dental problems. (North Americans of all ages now drink fifty-six gallons of soft drinks per person.) But fast-food chains also benefit when *children* drink more soft drinks; McDonald's sells more Coca-Cola than anyone else in the world. Soft-drink consumption was studied in a 1999 report entitled *Liquid Candy*, published by the Center for Science in the Public Interest, which determined that children are consuming obscene amounts of soft drinks. In 1978, the average male teen consumed about seven ounces of a brand-name soft drink per day;

as of this writing, male teens average about twenty-one ounces per day, and get 9 per cent of their calories just from soft drinks. Female teens consume about twelve ounces of soft drinks per day, which has doubled since the 1970s. Too many soft drinks also lead to calcium deficiencies, which can increase the risk of osteoporosis in adulthood, particularly in women.

In 1981, teens drank twice as much milk as soft drinks; today, this figure has reversed. Worse, about one-fifth of North American toddlers (one- and two-year-olds) now drink soft drinks in their bottles or no-spill cups. The shift in soft-drink consumption is significant. The supply of homogenized milk decreased from 25.5 gallons per capita per in 1970 to just 8.5 gallons in 1997, but soft-drink consumption rose from 24.3 gallons per capita to 53 gallons per capita during the same time frame.

PREVENTING CHILDHOOD OBESITY

North American children are considered the worst examples of childhood obesity. Children are now developing obesity-related diseases such as type 2 diabetes and high cholesterol, once diagnosed only in adults. Between the late 1970s and the early 1990s, the prevalence of childhood obesity has doubled (from 8 to 14 per cent in children six to eleven and from 6 to 12 per cent in teens). Fearing the same fate for their own children, many European countries have taken action. In 1992, Sweden banned all television advertising directed at children under twelve. Ads have similarly been banned from children's television programming in Norway, Belgium, Ireland, and Holland. Most countries look at North American children as an example of "what not to become."

In 1995, the American Academy of Pediatrics stated that advertising to children under eight was exploitative. Although companies doing the advertising assert that banning their ads would interfere with their freedoms, child health experts compare the peddling of junk food and fat to our children to peddling tobacco and alcohol to them. Preventing obesity in children means limiting their access to these ads.

THE OTHER SIDE OF MALNUTRITION: OVERNOURISHMENT

Nutrition experts also consider North Americans malnourished through *nutrient excess*. In the early twentieth century, public-health initiatives sought to lower rates of infectious diseases such as tuberculosis and diphtheria by improving nutrition. In 1900, life expectancy was under fifty; nutritionists encouraged people to eat a greater variety of foods, so that infectious diseases would not be made worse by malnutrition. Improvements in sanitation also led to fewer outbreaks of infectious diseases. By the 1970s, life expectancy rose to about seventy, which was considered a huge improvement. Foods became fortified with vitamins, such as iron, and school lunch programs were introduced, which helped to eliminate deaths among North American children from starvation and undernourishment. Then, as mentioned, once the food supply became more abundant, fortified, and accessible, sedentary living and a "diet of leisure" became the norm.

The seeds of sedentary life were already planted in the 1920s, as consumer comforts, mainly the automobile and radio, led to more driving, less walking, and more sedentary recreation. The Depression interrupted what was supposed to be prosperous times for everyone. It also intercepted obesity and all obesity-related diseases, as most industrialized nations barely ate enough to survive.

The Depression years, which ended in Canada when Britain declared war on Germany in 1939, combined with the six long years of war that followed, led to an unprecedented yearning for consumer goods such as cars, refrigerators, stoves, radios, and washing machines. As the boys marched home, they were welcomed with open arms into civilian bliss. By 1948, university enrollment had doubled, leading to an explosion in white-collar desk jobs and the commuter economy that exists today. The return of the veterans also led to an unprecedented baby boom, which would drive the candy, sweets, and junk-food markets for decades to come. Moreover, a sudden influx of money from Victory Bond investments and veterans' re-establishment grants coincided with the first payments of government pensions and family allowances. Never before had North Americans had so much money.

Manufacturers and packaged-goods companies were looking for better ways to compete and sell their products. The answer to their prayers arrived in the late 1940s with the cathode-ray tube: television. In the end, television would become the appliance most responsible for dietary decline and sedentary lifestyle as it turned into a babysitter that could mesmerize the baby-boom generation for hours.

THE DIET OF LEISURE

Naturally, after the war people wanted to celebrate. They gave parties, they drank wine. They smoked. They went to restaurants. More than ever before, our diets began to include more high-fat items, refined carbohydrates, sugar, alcohol, and chemical additives. And as people began to manage large families, easy-fix meals in boxes and cans were being manufactured in abundance and sold on television to millions.

The demand for the diet of leisure radically changed agriculture too. Today, 80 per cent of our grain harvest goes to feed livestock (those steaks for the barbecue). The rest of our arable land is used for other cash crops such as tomatoes, sugar, coffee, and bananas. Ultimately, cash crops have helped to create the modern Western diet, which contains an excessive amount of meat, eggs, dairy products, sugar, and refined flour.

Since 1940, chemical additives and preservatives in food have risen by 995 per cent. In 1959, the Flavor and Extract Manufacturers' Association of the United States (FEMA) established a panel of experts to determine the safety status of food flavorings to deal with the overwhelming number of chemicals that companies wanted to add to our foods. And one of the most popular food additives is monosodium glutamate (MSG), the sodium salt of glutamic acid, an amino acid that occurs naturally in protein-containing foods such as meat, fish, milk, and many vegetables. MSG is a flavor enhancer that researchers believe contributes a "fifth taste" to savory foods such as meats, stews, tomatoes, and cheese. It was originally extracted from seaweed and other plant sources to function in foods the same way as other spices or extracts. Today, MSG is made from starch, corn sugar, or molasses from sugar cane or sugar beets. MSG is produced by a fermentation process similar to that used for making products such as beer, vinegar, and yogurt. While MSG is labeled Generally Recommended as Safe (GRAS) by the U.S. Food and Drug Administration (FDA), questions about the safety of ingesting MSG have been raised because food sensitivities to the substance have been reported. This fact notwithstanding, the main problem with MSG is that it arouses our appetites even more. Widespread in our food supply, MSG makes food taste better. And the better food tastes, the more we eat.

Hydrolyzed proteins are also used as flavor enhancers. These are made by using enzymes to digest proteins chemically from soy meal, wheat gluten, corn gluten, edible strains of yeast, or other food sources. This process, known as hydrolysis, breaks down proteins into their component amino acids. Today, there are several hundred additive substances like these used in our food, including sugar, baking soda, and vitamins.

EATING MORE

Concerns about overnourishment have become a public-health crusade. In 1997, North American children got 50 per cent of their calories from added fat and sugar; only 1 per cent of children surveyed had a diet that resembled "variety" based on government nutritional guidelines such as Canada's Food Guide or the U.S. Food Pyramid; both Canada and the United States have almost parallel recommendations, stressing a diet that relies mostly on plant-based foods (grains, fruits, and vegetables), some dairy, less meat. Snack foods and sweets are not in these guidelines.

Another public-health irony is that, in spite of the over-abundance of food, many poor children in North America still do not have enough real food to eat; diets of poverty rely on cheaper, high-fat, overprocessed foods, which contribute to childhood obesity. In the late 1990s, roughly 3 million Canadians lived in poverty, and the majority were women; two-thirds of food-bank users were single mothers, while close to half a million children in this country – almost all in households headed by single mothers – were considered "food insecure" by Statistics Canada. According to the National Population Health Survey, half a million Canadians did not have enough money for food.

The diet-related medical costs for major obesity-related conditions, such as cardiovascular disease, diabetes, and certain cancers, total more than $70 billion. As a population, if we reduced our saturated fat intake by just 1 per cent, we could shave more than a billion dollars off health-care costs. The North American food supply is so abundant that we could feed everyone in the world twice over. Add to that an affluent society that can afford to buy "nice to have" foods versus "must have" foods, and you have a competitive marketplace for the food industry, which, by the way, was the industry that first labeled its end-user the "consumer" – based on (of course) how much of their product was literally consumed.

The food industry would not make money if it told us to eat less food. Therefore, it must tell us to eat more food. Marion Nestle, nutritionist and author of *Food Politics*, calls this the politics of "eat more," which dominate the food industry. To get us to eat more, food companies sometimes have to get us to eat more of one product instead of another. Distorted facts from various health studies may be combined with labeling to achieve this. Tomato sauce and ketchup producers tell us that lycopene in tomatoes will protect us from prostate cancer, so we are instructed to *eat more* of that and less of something else (more on lycopene in Chapter 8). We are told that if we *eat more* cereals with oats (no matter how much sugar and calories are mixed in with those oats), we'll prevent heart disease (more on that in Chapter 6). Studies looking at whether certain foods are of benefit to our health are frequently sponsored by food companies (more on that in Chapters 3 through 6).

We are also encouraged to eat more to get more value for our dollar. "Dollar meals," or getting an extra-large size of a particular product for "just a dollar/quarter/dime more," pushes us to eat more. Adding side products to the meal and selling it as a package also gets us to eat more. At many fast-food restaurants, it's easier (and faster) to buy the "Number 2" than to say, "I'll have a single cheeseburger with a salad, with dressing on the side." Usually, at fast-food restaurants less food *costs more* than the package deal with more food. (Does anyone *really* want the greasy hash browns that come with the McDonald's breakfast combo, or is just easier to order the combo to get the coffee for less?) Because of the way fast-food chains purchase commodities in bulk, they are able to offer value portions, which offer much larger portions for just a few cents more per person (translating into profit for the food companies). In the late 1950s, for example, adult-sized soft drinks were eight ounces; today, child-sized drinks at McDonald's are twelve ounces and a large soft drink is thirty-two ounces. A large fries at McDonald's in 1972 was three times smaller in portion size than the Super Size fries most people purchase today, which contain 610 calories and 29 grams of fat. If you ordered a regular hamburger, fries, and a twelve-ounce Coca-Cola, you would ingest 600 calories. Now, normal orders rarely involve regular hamburgers; most people order a Quarter Pounder with Cheese (440 calories), a Big Mac (580 calories), or a Big Xtra (600 calories). Add the Super Size fries and Super Size drink, and you're eating more.

In sit-down restaurants (particularly in the United States), the portions are enormous – often enough to feed four people. People feel obliged to finish the portions in order to get value for their dollar, or not to feel as though they're wasting money. Many restaurants now have No Sharing signs posted on menus, thus discouraging people from eating less. I visited one restaurant that offered a huge breakfast for just $2.99, allowing the customer to order from one to six eggs for the same price, with strict guidelines that one couldn't share (I hope this ensured that fewer people took advantage of the six-egg deal). All-you-can-eat buffets are popping up faster than you can say "all-u-can-eat." I have referred to these types of restaurants in the past as "obesity delivery systems." The value of the buffet outweighs the expense of ordering separately from the menu, so that almost everyone winds up at the buffet – at least twice – no matter how disciplined they try to be.

Companies have also found ways to market their "sub-products." Timbits – one of the most popular fast-food items sold in Canada – are marketed as "donut holes." Timbits were introduced in Canada in 1976 by the Tim Hortons chain (Dunkin' Donuts, the largest U.S.-based donut chain in North America, has a similar product called a Munchkin); today, people are encouraged to buy Timbits in bulk in a Snack Pack of twenty or a Family Pack of forty-five.

Pizza companies offer "dipping sauces" for the pizza crusts, which many people used to throw away. The dipping sauces thereby encourage people who would normally toss their crust, or not finish it, to *eat more*. Pizza companies now routinely offer an oxymoronic "dessert pizza," which, incredibly, has become popular. Consumers will order a pizza for dinner, which packs more than enough calories into it for the whole family. And then they "complete" their meal with a dessert pizza, in the form of large danishes or pies. There is an entire generation of children that think "dessert pizza" is a natural second course to regular pizza.

Currently, North Americans order roughly 3 billion pizzas a year from more than 60,000 pizzerias that are either chains (such as McDonald's-owned Donatos) or individually owned. One out of every six restaurants is a pizzeria; annual sales reach $30 billion and are topped only by hamburger sales. Although some nutritionists argue that pizza represents all food groups, many feel it is simply a high-calorie food no one needs. At Pizza Hut, three pieces of pizza have twelve grams of saturated fat, just under a third of the daily calorie limit from fat that Health Canada recommends the average Canadian should consume: 30 per cent or less, roughly 33 grams of fat per day for a 1,500-calorie diet.

LIFE IN THE FAST LANE

In Eric Schlosser's *Fast Food Nation*, he tells us how we "got here" – how we became a society ruled by fast-food chains that have infiltrated every aspect of our culture – to the detriment of our health or what he refers to as the "the McDonaldization of America" (a term coined by farm activist Jim Hightower). Indeed, the obesity epidemic hit North America when we began eating meals outside the home.

In 1900, women accounted for 21 per cent of the workforce, and married women less than 6 per cent. In 1999, women (married or not) accounted for 60 per cent of the workforce. By 2016, Statistics Canada predicts that the number of families run by single mothers will climb to roughly 1.6 million, up 60 per cent from today's 20 per cent. A small percentage of single mothers are widows, but the vast majority – 80 per cent – are divorced. This has led to a dependency on meals outside the home. Today, half our meals are prepared outside the home and 25 per cent are fast foods. We depend on prepackaged sandwiches, salads, entrees, and desserts. Within our supermarkets we now have salad bars, hot-food bars, barbecued or roasted chicken, and supermarket-prepared "home meal replacements." And then there are takeout foods.

A Canadian tradition is donuts and coffee in the morning, made popular by chains such as Tim Hortons, now one of North America's largest donut chains. Tim Hortons has more than 2,200 locations in Canada, and has now crossed the border into the United States with 160 locations. (It began with a single location in Hamilton, Ontario, started by Tim Horton, of National Hockey League fame.) Its expansion into the United States was made possible when, in 1995, it merged with Wendy's International, Inc. (Tim Hortons locations are now in Michigan, New York, Ohio, Kentucky, Maine, and West Virginia.)

In the U.S., the most successful donut chain in business history is Krispy Kreme, now in Canada, the United Kingdom, and Australia, with plans to go all over the world. Although Dunkin' Donuts is the largest donut chain in North America (with 3,600 locations), Krispy Kreme is predicted to outgrow Dunkin' Donuts, given its profit with just 292 locations as of this writing. In other words, the entire world may soon have access to the classic glazed Krispy Kreme donut, which packs 200 calories and 12 grams of fat.

If you look at the prices of grocery-bought convenience foods, such as frozen foods or supermarket-prepared "home meals," they're often not as cheap and predictable as fast food. That is why fast food proliferates. But even when we try to choose more-nutritious offerings, the hidden fat in fast food has made us fatter.

In surveys on dietary patterns conducted between 1970 and the late 1990s, people reported eating less fat; but dietary fat increased during that time by 25 per cent. U.S. Department of Agriculture (USDA) nutritionists accounted for these discrepancies by concluding that the fat was hidden. Although people thought they were "eating less fat," because they were choosing products they believed had less fat, they were actually eating more hidden fat within the products they had chosen.

With the exception of salads, fast food is prepared off-site and arrives at the chain in a frozen or freeze-dried state. We are not actually eating what we think we are. If you're a vegetarian, for example, you might be upset to learn that McDonald's fries are cooked in beef extract. Several lawsuits by vegetarians (particularly from India) followed this revelation. McDonald's publicly denied using beef extract in its franchises in India, but nonetheless settled the lawsuit in 2002, with a settlement fund that would go to vegetarian-related charities. As of November 2003, McDonald's still lists "natural flavor (beef source)" in its ingredients list on its Web site <www.mcdonalds.com>. Wendy's Grilled Chicken Sandwich also contains beef extract. Chicken McNuggets, introduced in 1983, are reconstituted chicken held together with stabilizers. They're breaded, fried, frozen, and then reheated. People select McNuggets, thinking that they're chicken and therefore lower in fat. But a Harvard study that analyzed the contents of McNuggets revealed that they were cooked in beef tallow and were more "beef" than fowl in the final analysis. Now McNuggets are cooked in vegetable oil, but beef extract is still used to make them. An order of Chicken McNuggets, a favorite menu item for children, actually has twice as much fat as a regular hamburger.

There are problems with hamburgers too. About 25 per cent of the ground beef used for hamburgers sold in fast-food chains comes from older and less healthy dairy cows, who can no longer produce healthy milk, along with free-range cattle raised specifically for food. Dairy cows frequently have antibiotic residue in their meat because of the antibiotics used in the dairy industry to prevent or to treat infections involving the cow's teats or udders. Meat from dozens of different cows is ground up together; one hamburger could come from several different animals, which can increase exposure to the notorious E. coli bacteria and is thought to have led to its rise.

Obesity rates go up everywhere fast food goes. Between 1984 and 1993, the number of fast-food chains in the United Kingdom doubled; so have its obesity rates. Britain, notorious for expensive, bad food and small portions by our standards, is now eating more fast food than any other country outside of North America. Other countries in the European Union, such as Italy, Spain, and France, lauded for their lower rates of obesity, have been studied by North Americans. What are they eating that accounts for this? Is it the olive oil? Is it the wine? (See Chapters 4 and 6.) But the truth may be simpler: *There are fewer fast-food chains in these regions.* Maybe it's not what they are eating, but what they are not, which is the answer to the French Paradox (see Chapter 6). Asian populations have also enjoyed the lowest obesity rates in the world among First World countries. But in China, obesity rates among teenagers has tripled since the 1990s, along with the rise of fast-food restaurants. Similarly, in Japan, obesity rates have doubled since the arrival of Ronald McDonald in 1971. Now, Japan is witnessing the first generation of thirty-something men who are obese.

Schlosser notes in *Fast Food Nation* that, in 1960, the typical North American ate only four pounds of frozen french fries per year; today, the typical North American consumes roughly forty-nine pounds of frozen fries per year – 90 per cent of which are purchased at fast-food restaurants. North Americans spent $6 billion on fast food in 1970; that number climbed to $110 billion by 2000 – more than North Americans spent on education, high-tech equipment cars, or any other item.

At least 25 per cent of the North American adult population enters a fast-food restaurant once a day. Unfortunately, most people don't go to fast-food chains to get the lighter fare; they are there to satisfy a craving for brand-name items they hate to love.

North Americans know – intrinsically – why they're getting fatter. The following Internet "chain joke," forwarded to hundreds of recipients by an anonymous author, speaks volumes about our collective knowledge about obesity trends.

The Good and Evil of Food

In the beginning God populated the earth with broccoli and cauliflower and spinach, green and yellow and red vegetables of all kinds, so man and woman would live long and healthy lives.

Then using God's great gifts, Satan created Ben and Jerry's and Krispy Kreme. And Satan said, "You want chocolate with that?"

And man said, "Yeah," and woman said, "And another one with sprinkles."

And they gained 10 pounds.

And God created the healthful yogurt that woman might keep the figure that man found so fair.

And Satan brought forth white flour from the wheat, and sugar from the cane, and combined them.

And woman went from size 2 to size 6.

So God said, "Try my fresh green salad."

And Satan presented Thousand Island dressing and garlic toast on the side. And man and woman unfastened their belts following the repast.

God then said, "I have sent you heart-healthy vegetables and olive oil in which to cook them."

And Satan brought forth deep-fried fish and chicken-fried steak so big it needed its own platter.

And man gained more weight and his cholesterol went through the roof.

God then brought running shoes so that his children might lose those extra pounds.

And Satan gave cable TV with a remote control so man would not have to toil changing the channels.

And man and woman laughed and cried before the flickering light and gained pounds.

Then God brought forth the potato, naturally low in fat and brimming with nutrition.

And Satan peeled off the healthful skin and sliced the starchy center into strips and chips and deep-fried them.

And man gained pounds.

God then created lean beef so that man might consume fewer calories and still satisfy his appetite.

And Satan created McDonald's and its 99-cent double cheeseburger. Then said, "You want fries with that?" and man replied, "Yeah! And Super Size 'em."

And Satan said, "It is good," and man went into cardiac arrest.

God sighed and created quadruple-bypass surgery.

So Satan created HMOs.

THE SKINNY

Obesity is an unhealthy state that increases our risks of many obesity-related diseases, such as type 2 diabetes and cardiovascular disease. Obesity is more prevalent in certain minority populations and is increasing at alarming rates in children. As we age, we become even less efficient at metabolizing calories too. Cumulative reductions in activity or energy expenditure can lead to a ten-pound weight gain each decade. So aging and longevity contributes to obesity as well.

Obesity is a weight determined to be medically unhealthy. Healthy weight ranges are now being distorted as a result of the rise in obesity, and a cultural "fear" of obesity. In many cases, obesity can be triggered by eating disorders that, essentially, mess up the body's normal metabolic system that protects against famine. By understanding obesity from this chapter, and learning about what is medically underweight in the next chapter, you can start to perceive what a healthy weight is more accurately for the balance of this book.

CHAPTER 2

EATING DISORDERS:

The Meaning of Fat and Thin

Although obesity may be a medically unhealthy state, so is the state of underweight, which in our North American culture is a self-induced, voluntary state. The majority of people who are underweight are women. Because of how they are socialized, most women are dissatisfied by what they see in the mirror. A third of the women in Canada believe they are overweight, even though their body weight is normal for their size, height, and age. Not surprising, 90 per cent of all eating disorders are diagnosed in women. In Canada, one in nine women between the ages of fourteen and twenty-five have an eating disorder, but this is certainly an under-reported problem. A *New York Times* poll as early as 1991 found that 36 per cent of girls aged thirteen to seventeen wanted to change their bodies; at least 10 per cent of girls aged fourteen and older suffered from eating disorders.

As a woman, I feel the social and cultural pressures to be thin. A few years ago, during a lecture, I was asked by a man to describe what it feels like to be a woman in our culture. My answer was:

"We get up in the morning and it begins. Continuous bombardment of beauty and fitness images from all forms of media. The result is that we are never beautiful enough, thin enough, or young enough to feel good about ourselves. Wherever we go, our appearance is watched and judged. Although women may be able to make peace with their appearance, and accept their bodies, it is next to impossible for most women to feel truly beautiful." The man was stunned and said, "This can't be true. It sounds so painful to be a woman." I then turned to the audience, where about one hundred women were sitting, and said, "If there's any woman in this room who feels what I just said is inaccurate, please raise your hand." No woman raised her hand. Instead, they quietly nodded to me, and some mouthed, "It's so true." Women's bodies are objects in our current culture, used to uphold, and impose, impossible standards of beauty. There is no woman who is immune to this powerful psychological attack. And so now we have created a culture in which women see their bodies as objects too. Experts in women's health and body image see a literal separation between mind, body, and spirit, sometimes known as mind-body dualism. These cultural standards of beauty play into the "low-fat" story in significant ways.

What women consider culturally "fat" and what the medical community considers "obese" do not match. People convinced they must adopt a diet that leads to weight loss may be under a delusion that they need to lose weight – a delusion that is promoted by the media through continuous bombardment of images of thin women and muscular, toned men. Once the habit of dieting begins, obesity can soon follow, as the body becomes more efficient with each calorie-restricting diet; it then takes less food to be as efficient as it was prior to the diet, which leads to further weight gain. This is what is widely known as yo-yo dieting, or weight cycling.

Many people with healthy body weights may be calling themselves "fat." Many people who are medically underweight may be calling themselves "normal" – or, too often, "fat" as well. And what our society deems "thin" may be what other cultures view as "starvation" or "malnutrition." Fat has become so feared in our culture that we have become what some experts call "fat phobic." People who define themselves as medically obese or as "fat" report what is now called "fat harassment." Our cultural attitude to obese people is out of control, and we are actually determining who is socially acceptable by body weight, rather than character. The result is that, for many people, self-esteem is completely tied to weight, creating a surge in "disordered eating" – from starvation and purging rituals to binge eating and yo-yo dieting. Weight is usually the most significant factor in body image, and body image affects both emotional and physical health. When someone has a negative body image, it can affect such things as food choices, physical activity, smoking, relationships, and even careers and education. It's been shown that people with poor body image are more prone to changing their weight in unhealthy, even dangerous, ways. Smoking, fad diets, starving and/or purging, or taking amphetamines or steroids are all common lifestyle habits adopted by people with poor body image. Children as young as ten are now dieting – and much of this is unnecessary dieting that leads to destructive behaviors in their teens and early adulthood. Depression is also more pronounced in people with poor body image.

Obesity, of course, is a problem for more than chronic dieters. For instance, sedentary living and overabundance of food, as well as fast-food advertising that targets children, has created an enormous increase in childhood obesity and obesity-related diseases in children – diseases that normally haven't been seen until adulthood. The purpose of this chapter is to explore how the fear of fat can lead to disordered eating and unhealthy weights on either side of the spectrum.

WHAT IS BODY IMAGE?

Body image is how we perceive our bodies, and how these perceptions make us *feel*. If we feel good about how we look, we have a positive body image; if we feel bad about how we look, we have a negative body image. Body image has nothing to do with someone's actual weight. People can be thin and have a negative body image; similarly, people may be obese and have a positive body image. Body image usually starts to form in childhood, when children with normal body weights can hear their parents express frequent concerns about their own weight and diet and begin to develop negative feelings about their own bodies. Other adults in a child's life, such as relatives, teachers, and coaches, can affect his or her body image. This is particularly true in sports. Other children may tease or bully them, which can affect body image and self-esteem. But the most influential external factor on a child's body image is the media – particularly in the case of girls.

WOMEN, WEIGHT, AND BEAUTY

In her book *The Body Project*, Joan Jacobs Brumberg, a professor of history and women's studies at Cornell, points out that a century ago a girl's sense of self was defined by her character, not her body. Today, girls and women use weight and beauty standards to define their identities; 53 per cent of North American girls are unhappy with their bodies, and by the time they reach the age of seventeen, the number jumps to a whopping 78 per cent.

A 2001 study published in the *Canadian Medical Association Journal* found that, of the 1,739 young Ontario girls aged twelve to eighteen who participated in the study, 27 per cent showed signs of eating disorders, 23 per cent reported being on a diet, 15 per cent reported binge eating, and 8.2 per cent were bulimic. Five per cent of the girls binged or purged at least twice a week. Some of the girls reported using diet pills, laxatives, or diuretics to lose weight.

According to nutrition experts from the University of Alberta, a "healthy weight" for a woman who is five feet, nine inches tall is anywhere from 135 to 189 pounds; for a woman who is five-feet-four, a healthy weight range is 115 to 164 pounds. *Prevention* magazine reports the average, healthy North American woman is about five-feet-three and weighs 152 pounds. Statistics from the fashion retail industry confirm this: 40 to 50 per cent of North American women are a size 14 or higher, while more than 25 per cent of fashion dollars are spent on sizes 16 and up. But the women portrayed in the media clearly do not match the reality of these demographics.

In contrast, the average model of five-feet-nine weighs just 110 to 115 pounds. Actress Julia Roberts, who is that height, weighs 121 pounds. Supermodel Heidi Klum, who is five-feet-nine-and-a-half, weighs even less – 119 pounds. Actresses who are billed as having more normal, full figures are underweight. Charlize Theron (five-feet-eleven and 135 pounds) should weigh 155; Gillian Anderson (five-feet-three and 115) should weight at least 120.

In 2001, a University of Toronto study looked at the impact of these media images on average women. When 188 women were shown pictures of thin models, they became depressed and angry.

Gallup poll surveys reveal that about 44 per cent of women diet to improve their health; 31 per cent of women polled say both health and appearance are a factor in their dieting. Yet the same survey revealed that just 22 per cent of women said they never worried about their weight. The same survey of men found that 46 per cent did not worry about their weight.

Results from a 1994 Mediamark Research, Inc. survey revealed that, at any given time, 40 per cent of women are trying to lose weight, 36 per cent are dissatisfied with their bodies, and 62 per cent are on diets even though they are not clinically obese. As for truly obese women, Mediamark found that 81 per cent of women whose average weight was 222 pounds were not dieting because they were convinced it wouldn't do any good.

Women are also more likely than men to view being over-weight as a personal failure, whereas men will blame excess weight on external lifestyle factors (such as long hours at work, long commutes, overreliance on fast food, etc.).

The beauty industry's impact on women's body image and dieting is so powerful that, in January 2002, YM magazine, which caters to teens, announced plans to stop publishing stories on dieting. The February 2002 issue of the magazine featured young models of varying body shapes, up to size 14, a trend that is now being seen in several women's magazines.

A 2002 University of Montreal study found that women living in middle-income and upper-income neighborhoods were 70 per cent more likely to be dissatisfied with their bodies than those who live in low-income neighborhoods. The lead study author pointed out that the easy availability of fashion magazines in more affluent homes was a significant factor in these results.

Many women also use exercise as a way to control their weight and purge themselves of calories. Although exercising is an essential component to improve overall health, and is imperative to offset our current sedentary living conditions, researchers are finding disturbing results when surveying reasons for exercising. Their habits often run counter to the goals of health; many abuse exercise to an unhealthy point.

In studies looking at exercise behavior in women, women often described their main goal of exercise as weight loss and toning their muscles to enhance their body shape and attractiveness. In other words, women often focus on the beauty benefits of exercise rather than the health benefits of exercise.

Studies also show a profound link between eating and exercise patterns in women. Women tend to think that, if they eat poorly, they must exercise; but also, if they exercise, they are "allowed" to eat. Generally, when women exercisers felt they ate too much, or ate unhealthy foods, they felt compelled to exercise to work off the excess calories. Women who routinely exercise view it as a punishment or compensation for their eating behaviors rather than as an activity that is part of a healthy lifestyle.

MEN AND BODY IMAGE

Men are not immune to body-image distortions either. Men tend particularly to abuse exercise and suffer more from what are termed "overuse injures." Men will frequently adjust their diet in order to appear bulkier and more muscular. For many men, this can lead them to take questionable diet supplements and even steroids. In recent years, reports of boys and men suffering from body-image distortions – seen in obsessions with "bulking up" and weightlifting – are on the rise. Media images of male models have, in turn, contributed to the problem. However, male actors of all sizes and shapes continue to be successful, and the media bombardment is not as intense for men at it is for women. Nonetheless, roughly 10 per cent of eating disorders are diagnosed in men and are expressed as the same diseases in men as they are in women. Young men in high school and college have been diagnosed with both anorexia and bulimia. Male sports most commonly associated with eating disorders in men are wrestling, distance running, horse racing, and bodybuilding.

The Canadian Centre for Ethics in Sports estimates that roughly 80,000 Canadian men are taking steroids to enhance their bodies. In the book *The Adonis Complex*, authors Dr. Harrison Pope, Dr. Roberto Olivardia, and Dr. Katharine Phillips report that males tend to suffer more from "muscle dysmorphia" – being unhappy with their muscular definition. Also described as "bigarexia" or "reverse anorexia," this is a condition where a man becomes addicted to bodybuilding. Whereas an anorexic never feels thin enough, a bigarexic never feels muscular enough. Men who are "bigarexic" will use exercise as their first strategy to "bulk up" and then use diet as a way to enhance their muscular build, such as taking supplements and steroids, but rarely eating healthily. Men tend to lack practical knowledge about nutrition, and can fall victim to the claims of nutriceuticals or can distort the messages they read about low-fat eating (see Chapters 1 and 4).

Men in their teens and twenties are the largest consumers of bodybuilding supplements. North Americans spent roughly $16.7 billion on supplements in 2000, according to the *Nutrition Business Journal*, and the most popular "growth" market is in "body image" supplements, which claim to help the mostly male users "bulk up" and add muscle tone. Some of these "bulking agents" are now in supermarkets.

In a 2001 U.S. survey of more than five hundred people at Boston-area health clubs, Pope found that 61 per cent of men used protein supplements in the past three years, 47 per cent said they had used creatine, 26 per cent said they had used ephedra (see Chapter 7), and 18 per cent had used andro. Most young men learn about supplements from their peers: teammates or friends at their gym. Steroid use tends to be highest among male teens aged fourteen to seventeen.

BELIEFS ABOUT THINNESS

There are also many socio-economic messages associated with a thin body. To some, a thin body sends the message of control. To be in control of our passions, our feelings, our emotions is something that is revered in our culture. A thin body is also masculine and less feminine, which implies a masculine emotional framework. A "successful" woman is a tall, thin, mannish woman who does not show evidence, on her body, of being female or of harboring reproductive organs. The beauty standard that we see on runways and in magazines reflects the masculinization of the female form. In Western culture, we have come to associate feminine curves with loss of control. The successful woman can look like a man because she *controls* her food intake. Some experts in eating disorders add that the control of internal impulses such as hunger are perceived as the conquering of animal instincts. The unsuccessful woman cannot control her food intake and therefore takes on the rounder shape, which is rejected by our society (although, admittedly, in other cultures, there are different beauty standards). So now controlling food is synonymous with self-control, self-discipline, and, ultimately, success – another facet of the power struggle. For many women, controlling the shape of their bodies gives them a sense of accomplishment. The irony is that a thin body can leave the impression of frailty or even illness.

BELIEFS ABOUT FATNESS

"Fat" people – especially women – in Western culture are considered to be out of control (although in other cultures fat women are nurturers, sensuous and life-giving). Perhaps one of the most powerful messages conveyed by fat women is that the fat woman feeds herself in a world where she is not supposed to feed her desires in any straightforward way.

The concept of "fat" has taken on other meanings – for women in particular. When a woman says she feels "fat," other women interpret that she feels vulnerable, unattractive, and depressed: the word *fat* encompasses all negative images and feelings for women.

FAT PHOBIA

The "meaning of fat" in our culture was actually measured in a study on fat phobia, an irrational fear of fat that experts define as "pathological," or unhealthy. Fat phobias are not unlike other prejudices, such as xenophobia (fear of different races or cultures) or homophobia (fear of homosexuals). In fat phobia, a person forms unfounded negative attitudes and stereotypes about fat people. This leads to harassment and unfair treatment of fat people within our society. Even the fat person can be infected by fat phobia. It is well documented that the social stigma of being fat is often a driving force behind eating disorders, fueled by a fear of fat so intense that women have expressed in studies and documentaries that they'd "rather be dead than fat."

Fat phobia tends to be stronger when the fat phobic (the person fearing the fat person) believes that their obesity was caused by the act of overeating rather than as a result of an underlying organic disease. One study from 1980 found that, when high-school girls were told that a fat girl was "fat" because of a thyroid problem, the fat girl was liked just as much as anyone else. But when the same girls were told a fat girl was "fat" because of her own tendency to overeat or to eat poorly, she was not well liked.

One of the best measurements of "the meaning of fat" in our culture comes from an actual Fat Phobia Scale, which was developed in 1984 by a researcher who asked people entering a motor-vehicle license bureau in a U.S. city to list adjectives describing people who are fat. Clinical facts were mixed with the descriptions from this survey to form a fifty-item scale currently used in studies that look at fat phobias. A 1997 study found, for example, that people who were average or underweight were more likely to have fat-phobic attitudes than those who were overweight. People younger than fifty-five were more likely to be fat phobic than people older than fifty-five; and, not surprisingly, women were more likely than men to be fat phobic. Another surprising finding is that the more education a person has, the more fat phobic they are. They appear to believe that, because of information about diet and nutrition, there is no "excuse" any more to be fat. People who come from lower socio-economic backgrounds or who have less education are less fat phobic. This has to do with the fact that lower socio-economic cultures have less access to nutritious, fresh foods and to gyms. Medical professionals on the whole were less fat phobic, because they know about what truly leads to obesity, although anecdotal evidence points to some terrible fat harassment and bias towards fat patients from health-care providers.

Those who revealed prejudice against fat people in the 1997 fat-phobia study viewed fat people as undisciplined, inactive, and unappealing; they viewed overeating and lack of willpower as unattractive. They also viewed fat people as having emotional and psychological problems. Fat phobia is not only more prevalent among women than men, but women will voice their fears of fat more openly to other fat women.

FAT HARASSMENT

Fat women report that they often receive insults disguised as "concern" from thinner women. Thinner women will make comments on a fat woman's food choices in public; they will say things such as, "Are you sure you need to eat all that?" to a fat female they don't even know. "Helpful" advice offered at the grocery store to a fatter customer includes: "There's a low-fat version of that"; "Have you tried the low-fat or 1% brand?" Rude and disdainful glances into fatter women's shopping carts are made frequently, especially if high-fat snacks are in the cart.

Women who have gained weight after childbirth also report being "harassed" for their weight gain.

Fat harassment comes out in the workplace as well. Overweight white women were found to be paid less than comparably qualified normal-weight white women, according to a University of Michigan study done for the National Bureau of Economic Research in the 1990s. Women of average weight were found to be paid 7 per cent more. An eight-year study published in the *New England Journal of Medicine* revealed that fat people earn roughly $7,000 less than those with similar training in comparable jobs.

People who are morbidly obese (see Chapter 1) report how frequently they are asked for an interview, based on their qualifications on paper, but are routinely denied the job because (they presume) of their appearance. One survey conducted by the National Association for the Advancement of Fat Acceptance (NAAFA) found that 40 per cent of men and 60 per cent of women stated that – although difficult to prove legally – they had not been hired for a job due to weight. Lack of advancement or promotion within stagnant jobs was also reported.

Fat people also report on-the-job harassment from employers and co-workers. Women are frequently told they are sloppy or look unprofessional in their performance reviews. Yet attractive large-sized clothing is expensive and difficult to find. Shopping for clothing frequently exposes a fat woman to harassment and unwelcome comments from salespeople.

Fat people, by routinely being denied access to normal social activities such as shopping for decent clothing, report feeling stigmatized, as though they are viewed as lazy, stupid, ugly, incompetent, filthy, greedy, sexless, and/or desperate for sex and unattractive; they further report, based on their experiences, being perceived as hoarding food, being helpless or weak, taking up too much space, straining health-care resources, and lacking self-control.

In the United States, some fat people are automatically denied health coverage by medical plans, simply based on their weight. Doctors routinely dismiss legitimate health complaints, attributing them to being overweight. One female journalist who self-identifies as "fat" reported that her doctor blamed her pain from a twisted ankle on her weight. The doctor-on-call refused to take an X-ray, saying that, because she was fat and "probably" had diabetes (without checking, in fact), her foot would probably "fall off anyway," so why waste an X-ray. He further informed her that her ankle would heal if she lost weight.

There are more invisible forms of harassment fat people report, which have to do with squeezing their body sizes into a world not built for them (similar complaints are found amongst people with disabilities). For example, narrow seating in theaters, on planes, and in restaurants make things difficult for someone who is fat. (I recall an incident on a plane, in which a heavy man seated next to me broke the seat, became terribly embarrassed, and had to endure a broken seat for the remainder of the flight.) There are also nasty comments such as: "If you're fat enough to take up two seats, you should pay for two seats." Narrow aisles in stores, narrow bathroom stalls, narrow and squat car seats, and tiny changing rooms are constant problems. Accessories such as glasses, watchbands, hats, socks, jewelry, and so on, made to average standards, never fit.

Many women coming of age see how fat women are treated in our culture and grow so fearful of becoming fat and so conscious of their bodies that they frequently adopt disordered eating behaviors as a prophylactic measure to avoid that fate. Indeed, most women begin dieting to "prevent" becoming fat rather than dieting when they are, in fact, overweight.

DISORDERED EATING

Distorted body image, a fear of fat (or fat phobia), as well as distorted assumptions associated with thinness are the social building blocks to eating disorders and, more accurately, disordered eating, which includes binge eating disorder (BED).

Eating disorders affect women ten times more frequently than men and, in the overall population, affect roughly 5 per cent of adolescent girls (2 per cent suffer from anorexia, 3 per cent suffer from bulimia). However, the number of people suffering from BED is not calculated in these figures, since many who binge are "counted" by epidemiologists as simply obese, without consideration that the cause of their obesity is a disordered way of eating, usually fueled by feelings of low self-esteem connected to their body weight. Although Chapter 1 discusses obesity at length, this section explains some of the psychological factors and criteria that go into disordered eating.

Research on anorexia and bulimia reveals that about 60 per cent of anorexics become bulimic when they cannot endure starving themselves. According to the World Health Organization, the mortality rate among those diagnosed with anorexia is 15 per cent. According to a SmartGirl Web site survey, <www.smartgirl.org>, almost half of all respondents aged between ten and twenty said they knew someone with an eating disorder.

DEFINING EATING DISORDERS

Anorexia and bulimia are eating disorders fueled by body-image distortions and fat phobia; binge eating disorder is fueled by the emotional comfort associated with eating.

Anorexia Nervosa: Food Refusal. The person suffering from anorexia is not willing or able to keep a healthy body weight. S/he has a desire to control food and is frightened of "fat" or becoming fat, even when the body is in a state of starvation that threatens survival. Physical signs of anorexia include a weight that is 15 per cent below the ideal weight, no menstruation (in girls who do menstruate, menstruation stops; in girls too young to menstruate, it never starts), hair loss, dry skin, and a feeling of being too cold. Behaviors include cutting food into tiny pieces before eating, chewing for long periods of time, strange rituals revolving around food, and use of loose clothing (to hide the body).

Bulimia Nervosa: Food Bingeing and Purging. Someone suffering from bulimia will binge and purge. In a binge, s/he can consume thousands of calories at one sitting, and purge through vomiting, laxative and diuretic abuse, or exercise abuse. The binge is followed by feelings of depression and panic; the purge is followed by feelings of relief and comfort. Binge-and-purge cycles can badly damage the digestive system and affect vital organs; gastrointestinal disorders plague bulimics. Someone has bulimia if s/he binges at least twice a week for a period of three consecutive months, self-induces vomiting after eating, abuses laxatives or diuretics, goes on a drastically reduced diet after a period of eating, or exercises excessively on a regular basis. Physical signs of bulimia can include significant fluctuations in weight, dental problems as a result of repeated vomiting, and swelling of the salivary glands. Behaviors of bulimics can include chewing food and spitting it out, drinking large amounts of liquid to feel full or to provoke vomiting, fasting, eating quickly, barely chewing before swallowing, hiding when eating, and stealing food.

Binge Eating Disorder (BED): Compulsive Overeating. Someone suffering from BED derives comfort from eating, which helps to quell deep feelings of inadequacy and low self-esteem. In this case, the sufferer binges just as someone with bulimia does, but does not purge. S/he will binge to excess. The result is obesity and obesity-related health problems such as cardiovascular disease and type 2 diabetes (see Chapter 2). Behaviors of binge eaters include eating when they're not hungry, eating in secret or with "eating friends," appearing in public to be a professional dieter who's in control (but who never loses weight), buying cakes or pies as "gifts" and having them wrapped to hide the fact that they will be eaten later, presenting a "pristine" kitchen with only the "right" foods, and anticipating with pleasure when they can eat alone.

Eating disorders are addictions. The drug in anorexia is the control the anorexic feels over food. In bulimia, the binge is tremendously comforting and addictive; the purge is also comforting, as it gives back control. In BED, the food is the drug; the act of eating is tremendously satisfying and comforting. In all three disorders, the preoccupation with food prevents the sufferers from thinking about other problems in their lives.

FOOD AND FEELINGS

Many people will substitute food for other things that are missing in their lives, such as sexual satisfaction, love, or other sensuous aspects of life. On the flip side, when people feel their lives are out of control, they may use food as a way to regain control, or regain feeling, which is what is behind manipulating body sizes through food refusal or purging behaviors (for thin bodies) or overeating behaviors (for large bodies). Most research on the emotional connections to food and feelings has been done with women, since they suffer ten times more from eating disorders than men. (Of course, many of the findings are transferable to men with eating disorders.) One celebrity example can be seen in the late Princess of Wales, Diana, whose episodes of what she called "rampant bulimia – if there is such a thing" compensated for an existence in which she felt she was unable to express any of her feelings. Diana described the food in her bingeing episodes as being like a "warm hug." When women control their food intakes through starvation or purging, they are controlling their feelings – both negative and positive.

Research on bulimia and anorexia reveals that people with these eating disorders are usually overachievers in other aspects of their lives and view excess weight as an announcement to the world that they are "out of control." This view becomes more distorted as time goes on, until the act of eating food in public (in bulimia) or at all (in anorexia) is perceived to be equivalent to a loss of control.

In anorexia, the person's emotional and sensual desires are channeled through food. These desires are so great that the anorexic fears that, once she eats, she'll never stop since her appetite/desires will know no natural boundaries; the fear of food drives the disease. Many experts also see this eating disorder as an addiction to perfection.

Most of us find it easier to relate to the bulimic than the anorexic. Bulimics express their loss of control through bingeing. Bulimics then purge to regain their control. There is a feeling of comfort for bulimics in both the binge and the purge. Bulimics are sometimes referred to as "failed anorexics," because they'd starve if they could. Anorexics, however, are masters of control. They never break.

Some view the anorexic woman as the "nutritional virgin." In the past, women exhibited starving, bingeing/purging behaviors when it came to sex. The "sexual anorexic" was the virgin who denied herself sexual desires but at the same time was preoccupied with them. The "sexual bulimic" was the "slut" who slept around and was made to feel very guilty about indulging her desires; she may have even purged the consequences through a "coat hanger" abortion. Now that sexuality is allowed, however, the battle of desires is fought not in the back seat of a convertible but in the kitchen. In the past, young girls learned to repress their sexual appetites because of the consequences (pregnancy, becoming unmarriageable); today, young girls learn to repress their literal appetites because they fear similarly negative social consequences.

By starving themselves, women can also make their flesh disappear. Some who study the problem believe that, when these women are thin, and have no flesh, their twisted perception is that they can stop their feelings and desires. By having bodies, they feel their lives – hunger and desire (for food or sex), fullness and frustration, pleasure and pain. But when they are flat figures – images instead of bodies – or "no-body bodies," the desires vanish. Women tend to find it safer to live outside their bodies rather than inside. Research consistently shows, for example, that young women are far more concerned with how people see their bodies than with what they are seeing from within their bodies. Many girls and women talk about how their feelings make them look, rather than how they make them feel. In essence, the current beauty standard denies women their active desires.

THE SKINNY

As the obesity rates go up, so does fear of obesity, which is calculated according to a body mass index (Chapter 1). Actual obesity does not match what many perceive to be "obesity" or "fat" in the mirror. Thus, people who are of normal weights or are underweight may unnecessarily begin very low-calorie diets, triggering mechanisms within the body that make it more efficient at storing calories as fat. Fear of obesity can be responsible for weight gain in these cases, and for severe eating disorders. People who suffer from eating disorders will also distort nutritional information; they will take popular concepts surrounding health and fitness, for example, and twist them into misconstrued facts that support their disorders. Anorexics will take information about low fat to an extreme, believing that all fat and calories are harmful. Both anorexics and bulimics will take information about exercise to an extreme and abuse physical activity, distorting the amount of exercise required to burn calories. At the same time, compulsive overeaters will absorb information about the failure of diets, or other nutritional information, and will overeat the "right foods." Distorting nutritional information is easy when you understand how contradictory are the messages we receive about food. These messages will be discussed throughout the following chapters, as distorting nutritional information and health is particularly confusing when cancer and low fat are concerned.

CHAPTER 3

DIET, FAT, AND CANCER

There are legitimate reasons for lowering body fat that have to do with lowering your risk of certain diseases, including cancer. This chapter explores what we absolutely know about the role diet plays in cancer incidence, as well as what we suspect but can't prove about diet and cancer. The most comprehensive summary of diet and cancer done to date was a 1997 report entitled *Food, Nutrition and the Prevention of Cancer: A Global Perspective*, commissioned and published by the U.K.'s World Research Cancer Fund (WCRF) and the American Institute for Cancer Research (AICR). It contains the work of many organizations and individual experts, and was designed to address the primary prevention of cancer from a global perspective. All aspects of food and nutrition likely to reduce or to increase cancer risk were reviewed. The panel assembled for the report agreed on a consistent method to assess the various types of scientific evidence. This report was an exhaustive review of the scientific and other expert literature published between the late 1970s and late 1990s, linking foods, nutrition, food processing, dietary patterns, and related factors with the risk of human cancers worldwide.

In Canada, the *Report of the Ontario Task Force on the Primary Prevention of Cancer*, published in 1995, represented a broad range of scientific as well as public perspectives – including those of cancer survivors – about the primary prevention of cancer. The task force was chaired by Dr. Anthony Miller, chair of the Department of Preventive Medicine and Biostatistics at the University of Toronto. A key Ministry of Health representative was Dr. Les Levin, a supporter of primary cancer prevention and service adviser on cancer policy for the ministry. The report was facilitated by the former director of the University of Toronto's Centre for Health Promotion, Dr. Irving Rootman. An interdisciplinary team of environmental scientists, oncologists, and activists from across Ontario put thousands of hours into this report, which was also based on an exhaustive review of existing science. In 2001, I published *Stopping Cancer at the Source*, a book that explained many of the task force recommendations in plain language, and added to it from my own literature review of cancer risks. All of these reviews were used to form the content of this chapter with respect to nutrition, diet, fat, and cancer risks. This chapter is designed to help you sort out what to take seriously – or lightly – in the news when you hear: "A new study says . . ."

ASSESSING YOUR CANCER RISK

We're all born with a big "basement light switch" wired for potential diseases, including certain cancers. At birth, all of those switches are off. As we age and indulge in certain diets, habits, or activities or are exposed to certain toxins through work or lifestyle choices, these switches can be turned on. Nobody knows which switches are being turned on at certain points. All we can do is try to eliminate the triggers that can change our switches from off to on. Any cancer that is linked to the following can be stopped at the source through lifestyle modification that involves a combination of health-enhancement, risk-avoidance, or risk-reduction tactics such as:

- smoking, substance or alcohol abuse;
- poor high-fat, low-nutrient diets; and
- sedentary or inactive lifestyle.

Other environmental factors would be exposure to the sun and to certain infectious agents, as well as environmental toxins in the home or workplace. I discuss these factors at length in *Stopping Cancer at the Source*, but in this book I have limited the discussion to diet and the role of dietary fat in cancer incidence.

UNDERSTANDING RISK FACTORS

In order to practice health enhancement, risk avoidance, or risk reduction, you need to understand what is really meant by the phrase *risk factors*. What does it mean when you're told you're "at risk" for a particular cancer – or any other disease? The answer is: a few things, depending on the adjective that precedes the word *risk*.

When trying to understand risk factors, having a degree in actuarial science helps. That's because there is a world of difference between absolute, cumulative, relative, and attributable risk. Absolute risk means that the cancer rate is counted in numbers of cases occurring within a group of people. When you hear that in the town of Anywhere, "50 out of 100,000 people died last year of a particular cancer," this is absolute risk. The official definition of absolute risk is "the observed or calculated probability of an event in a population under study." So this can be a hypothetical or real population; it's just not relative to any *other* population.

Cumulative risk just means "added up." It's a risk per unit of time added up over X units of time, such as a lifetime or a given time frame that a study ran (i.e., two years or ten years). It can be an estimate or the experiences of a real group of people – but it will be an average of the experience of that group. So when you see "cumulative risk factors," it is a "guess" of risk based on a number of factors that may include mortalities from a particular cancer in a given area, in a certain age group, or in people who share your medical history. So cumulative risk is not based on you personally but on estimates. It's like betting on a horse race. You look at the ages of the horses, the histories, the breeding, the jockeys, and where the race is being run, and you come up with odds. When you read that "one in eight people over a lifetime" will get a particular cancer, this is a cumulative risk: an average, not an absolute. The problem with a statement like that is that it tends to underestimate risk in some, while overestimating risk in others. For example, not everyone on a high-fat diet will get cancer; not everyone on a low-fat diet will prevent cancer.

Then there's relative risk, which is based on comparing two populations. When people who eat large amounts of fat are at greater risk for certain cancers than people who have low-fat diets, this refers to relative risk. It directly compares a population that has one type of risk factor to a population that has a different risk factor. It basically compares risk in situation A with risk in situation B (which is usually a standard or constant, such as "no-risk factor").

But this doesn't mean that people who eat large amounts of fat cannot alter their diets, or people who smoke cannot quit smoking. When you speak of risk that can be reduced, prevented, or altered through behavior (like quitting smoking or dieting), you're now talking about *modifiable risk* because it is under voluntary control. This is different from a "risk marker," such as family history, which cannot be modified. It is also different from *attributable risk*, which refers to a component of one's risk attributable either to a modifiable risk factor such as diet or a risk marker such as family history.

Not all cancers can be linked to an absolute cause, either. For example, breast cancer is not like lung cancer. With lung cancer, we know that at least 70 per cent of those who develop it smoke. Therefore, you can absolutely say that smoking causes lung cancer, a cancer that kills more people each year than any other cancer. You can't name one main cause of breast cancer, however. All you can do is count up the people who are diagnosed with the disease, examine the kinds of lifestyles or family histories they have that may be different from those of people without breast cancer, and analyze the effects of each type of difference.

What most of us have been bombarded with since the 1970s are the reports of *known* risk factors for certain cancers, which refers to factors proven to increase the risk of certain cancers, such as tobacco. It's important to understand that many of the known risks are conflicting and often controversial. While one study suggests that this or that increases your risk of some cancer, another study may suggest the contrary.

Statistics are tricky. If odds are less than one to twenty of something being found *by chance*, it's said to be "statistically significant." Therefore, even if a certain characteristic, such as eye color, makes absolutely no difference to anybody's chance of getting a particular cancer, for every twenty studies or comparisons done on this characteristic, only one of those studies will show a "significant" departure from the conclusion of "no difference" between cases of people with a particular cancer and the control group (people without that particular cancer). When you see or hear "statistically significant" in the media, remember that it may mean "we found this purely by chance," even though the media may be going wild. The bottom line is that you have to be careful not to jump to conclusions when you hear breaking news about a new risk. That said, it's important to understand that no single risk factor, such as age or diet, can be interpreted as an *absolute cause* of most cancers. There are many lifestyle changes you can make to significantly lower your risks. In addition, understanding the environmental impact on many cancers will help you put these risks in perspective.

Another final distinction is the difference between *association* and *causation*. When you read a statement like "Men with prostate cancer were found to eat more fat than men without prostate cancer," this means association. It does not mean that dietary fat causes prostate cancer. When you read the sentence "Smoking causes lung cancer," this is an example of causation.

RISK CO-FACTORS

Cancer risk is usually not dependent on a single factor; it is multi-factorial. When assessing the extent to which diet and fat play a role in cancer, the following co-factors can increase risk:

1. Age: The risk of many cancers is largely age-related because so much cancer is dependent on our behaviors throughout our lives. The tendency is for most cancers to strike after age forty-five.
2. Bad habits: If you smoke, drink an excessive amount of alcohol, or abuse illegal drugs, your risk of getting cancer will probably be higher than it is for people who don't do these things.
3. Genetics: There are certain cancers to which some people may be genetically predisposed, given certain environmental triggers, such as diet. At the same time, some cancers may be genetic without such triggers. Genetic screening and genetic testing can provide meaningful information in some cases, and less meaningful information in others; but if you know you're genetically "wired" for a certain cancer, modifying diet and lifestyle may help to reduce the likelihood of getting a particular cancer.
4. Poor exercise habits: Sedentary living breeds ill health and is associated with higher rates of many cancers.
5. Industrialization: Who gets cancer largely depends on where people live. Many cancers are "regional." For example, industrialized countries have much higher rates of certain cancers than underdeveloped countries, and these are linked to various pollutants.
6. Occupational hazards: A woefully inadequate body of knowledge exists about workplace carcinogens. In urban centers, residents are exposed to a wide array of carcinogens in their workplaces, but there is only clear evidence of the cancer-causing potential for nine substances (known as the Noxious Nine): benzene, diesel exhaust, polycyclic aromatic hydrocarbons, perchloroethylene, dioxin, pesticides,

metalworking fluids, methylene chloride, and asbestos. As for the rest of the long list of suspected carcinogens, researchers point to the need for "more research in the future." The most important investigation into workplace carcinogens is the ongoing review process at the International Agency for Research on Cancer in Lyon, France. This material is reproduced in *Stopping Cancer at the Source.*

DIET AND CANCER

Diet plays an enormous role in cancer risk. One of the most significant ways in which diet affects cancer risk is socio-economic. Both diets of poverty and privilege are associated with different cancers.

Poor nutrition is associated with higher incidence of and mortality from the following:

- stomach cancer (poor diet);
- lung cancer in men (smoking, which is often a co-factor in poor diet);
- cervical cancer (smoking is associated with higher rates of cervical cancer, and many women start smoking to control weight); and
- cancers of the mouth, pharynx, larynx, and esophagus (related to smoking and poor diet).

Higher-income groups don't get away scot-free, because there are certain cancers that are linked to "luxury" or "opportunity" such as higher-fat diets, which usually are seen with less physical activity (more cars). Higher-fat diets are associated with a higher incidence of and mortality from the following:

- breast cancer;
- prostate cancer; and
- colon cancer in men.

As you look at this list, it's easy to see how lifestyle habits affect certain groups. "Wealthy" cancers – colon, breast, prostate – could be partially caused by high-fat (or privileged) diets and too much driving and not enough physical activity, as well as skin cancer, due to too much vacation and leisure time in the sun. So when it comes to tracking the incidence of disease, it's important to remember that socio-economic differences often bring with them corresponding differences in health-related behaviors, such as smoking, alcohol consumption, and poor eating habits. Reducing the much higher rates of smoking among economically disadvantaged groups is perhaps our biggest task in bringing about a reduction in socio-economic inequities in health status. All lifestyle behaviors have to be looked at in the context of the social, economic, environmental, and political factors that motivate them and that act, in many cases, as barriers to the maintenance of good health.

WHAT YOU EAT AND DRINK

Obesity is strongly associated with several cancers, most notably kidney, endometrial, breast, colon, rectal, and gallbladder cancers. Body fat also increases cancers that are estrogen-dependent because fat cells make estrogen; the estrogen your body produces can make a cancer cell thrive. Estrogen-dependent cancers include breast, endometrial, and colon cancers. Thus, in addition to the other health risks associated with obesity, which are discussed in previous chapters, these cancers can be added to the list.

Even putting obesity aside, human and animal studies point to the same conclusion: Diet can both increase and reduce your risk of cancer. Dietary risk factors have been linked to a number of common cancers, including stomach, breast, colon, and prostate. Protective factors, especially those derived from plant foods such as fruits and vegetables, have been associated with reduced risk of many cancers. Most cancer experts agree that next to smoking, diet is the second leading modifiable cause of cancer.

WHAT THE STUDIES SHOW

Overall, studies show that people who consume large amounts of dietary fat and meat are more likely to develop, and die from, breast and colon cancer, as well as cancers of the ovary, kidney, endometrium (lining of the uterus), and lung. One of the problems with many epidemiological studies is that, while they indicate trends in particular groups of people, they can't tell us how and why each individual's diet affects him or her. There are so many other factors that can affect diet, including childbearing patterns, genetics, activity levels, and stress.

Studies measuring dietary links to cancer are fraught with complications. It's sometimes hard for study participants to remember their food intake accurately, even if they're keeping journals. And since there are many components within one item, such as a hamburger (starches, proteins, chemicals in condiments, vegetables on top of the hamburger, and cooking method), even a superb record from a study participant can be hard to analyze.

Just how much cancer is linked to poor diet? Estimates vary from 15 to 75 per cent, but in light of more recent studies, it looks as if we're hovering at 30 per cent, which is very significant. That said, based on current studies, some cancers can absolutely be linked to diet, such as colon and rectal cancer, while the link between diet and other cancers still remains foggy, such as the link between diet and breast cancer.

The following is what we know so far about various food groups and cancer risk. The term *convincing evidence* means there is enough evidence to demonstrate an absolute link; the term *probable* refers to a strong link; the term *possible* refers to an established link; the term *insufficient evidence* means a link has been made in the published studies but not enough backup from other studies clearly demonstrates that the link is serious enough to be considered; the term *no relationship* means just that: there is no study published in the literature showing a link exists or a study has revealed that a suspected link is not there.

Carbohydrates

It is possible that fiber can decrease the risk of colon, rectum, pancreatic, and breast cancer. It is also possible that refined starchy diets, which are usually high in salt, can increase the risk of stomach, colon, and rectal cancers. It is possible that whole-grain cereals decrease the risk of stomach cancer, while refined cereals can increase the risk of esophageal cancers. There is insufficient evidence, however, to demonstrate that whole-grain cereals can decrease the risk of colon cancer.

Fats

There is no relationship so far between cholesterol and breast cancer, or between "good fats" (see Chapter 8) and breast cancer, either. It is possible, however, that cholesterol levels can increase the risk of lung cancer and pancreatic cancer, but there is insufficient evidence to demonstrate that cholesterol can increase the risk of endometrial cancer.

It is possible that diets high in total fat, which contribute to obesity and body size, can increase the risk of lung, colon, rectum, breast, and prostate cancers. There is insufficient evidence to demonstrate a link between total fat intake and ovary, endometrial, and bladder cancers. It is possible that diets high in saturated fats can increase the risk of lung, colon, rectum, breast, endometrium, and prostate cancers. There is insufficient evidence to demonstrate a link between saturated fat intake and ovarian cancer.

Vegetables and Fruits

There is convincing evidence that a diet rich in fruits and vegetables decreases the risk of mouth and pharynx, esophageal, lung, stomach, colon, and rectal (vegetables only) cancers. There is probable evidence that vegetables and fruits can decrease the risk of larynx, pancreatic, breast, and bladder cancers; and possible evidence that fruits and vegetables can decrease the risk of cervical, ovarian, endometrial, thyroid, liver (veggies only), prostate (veggies only), and kidney (veggies only) cancers. There are very few studies done on legumes and cancer risk, and so there is no good evidence about which legume to consume to reduce cancer risk.

Meat, Poultry, Fish, and Eggs

Today, it is probable that a diet high in red meat increases the risk of colon and rectal cancer; and possible that a diet high in red meat increases the risk of pancreatic, breast, prostate, and kidney cancers. It is possible that a diet high in eggs increases the risk of colon and rectal cancers, but there is insufficient evidence to support that eggs can increase the risk of pancreatic or ovarian cancers. There is insufficient evidence to demonstrate that fish can protect against breast and ovarian cancers, and no relationship between poultry and breast cancer; fish and colon or rectal cancer; eggs and kidney or bladder cancers.

Milk and Dairy Products

The evidence surrounding milk, dairy, and cancer links specifically is very low. It is possible that too much milk and dairy can increase the risk of prostate and kidney cancers. See also "Fats," where most of the studies focus on saturated fats, based on animal fats. See also "Vitamins"; many studies on vitamin D, which is in milk and dairy products, have been done.

Minerals from Various Food Groups

We know it's possible that selenium decreases lung cancer; there is insufficient evidence to demonstrate that selenium decreases stomach, liver, or thyroid cancers or that vitamin D decreases colon and rectal cancers. It is probable that not enough iodine increases the risk of thyroid cancer, and possible that too much iodine increases the risk of thyroid cancer. There is insufficient evidence to show that iron increases the risk of liver, colon, or rectal cancers, and there's no relationship between colon cancer and intake of calcium and selenium.

Vitamins from Various Food Groups

There's a reason why I stress here and in Chapter 4 how important it is to have a diet rich in fruits and vegetables: it's the vitamins in those foods that are an important part of decreasing cancer risk. So far, it is probable that carotenoids (which include the plant precursors of vitamin A) decrease the risk of lung cancer, and vitamin C decreases the risk of stomach cancer. It is possible that carotenoids decrease the risk of esophageal, stomach, colon, rectum, breast, and cervical cancers, and vitamin C decreases the risk of mouth, pharynx, esophageal, lung, pancreatic, and cervical cancers. It is also possible that vitamin E decreases the risk of lung and cervical cancers. There is insufficient evidence to demonstrate, however, that carotenoids can decrease larynx, ovarian, endometrial, or bladder cancers; that vitamin C decreases larynx, colon, rectum, breast, or bladder cancers; that retinol decreases bladder cancer; that vitamin E decreases colon or rectal cancers; or that folate and methionine decrease colon or rectal cancers.

There is no relationship between vitamin C and prostate cancer; retinol and lung, stomach, breast, or cervical cancers; vitamin E and stomach and breast cancers, or folate and cervical cancer.

Diet and Colon Cancer

Of all the studies done on the link between cancer and dietary fat, the strongest connections can be made between high-fat diets and colon cancer. In other words, people who consume high quantities of fat have higher rates of colon cancer; people who consume low quantities of fat have lower rates of colon cancer.

As for fiber, studies show that people who consume high quantities of fiber have lower rates of colon cancer; people who consume low quantities of fiber have higher rates of colon cancer. In addition, people who have regular bowel movements have lower incidences of colon cancer than people who are chronically constipated. It's safe to say that by lowering fat and increasing fiber, you can possibly reduce your risk of colon cancer. Canadian experts believe that, by following a low-fat, high-fiber diet, you may be able to avoid 90 per cent of all stomach and colon cancers and 20 per cent of gallbladder, pancreatic, mouth, pharynx, and esophageal cancers.

Diet and Breast Cancer

We know that breast cancer rates are four to seven times higher in North America than in Asia. When Asian women move to North America, their risk doubles over a decade and they seem to acquire breast cancer at North American rates after several generations. We don't know what accounts for this difference. Is it diet – are we eating something we shouldn't or are they eating some foods when in Asia that we should? For example, Japanese diets average roughly 15 per cent calories from fat; North American diets average about 40 per cent calories from fat. The traditional low-fat Japanese diet of rice, vegetables, and fish is light-years away from the meat and high-fat diet of North Americans.

The Japanese diet is also rich in plant estrogens (called phytoestrogens), which are found in tofu. Phytoestrogens act as weak estrogens, which interfere with ordinary estrogen production. And since estrogen seems to promote breast tumors, anything that interferes with estrogen should, theoretically, cut the risk. Some studies suggest that phytoestrogens may be associated with lower rates of breast cancer and less severe menopausal symptoms. Phytoestrogens are found in a variety of fruits and vegetables, including all soybean and linseed products, apples, alfalfa sprouts, split peas, and spinach.

Perhaps culture is a large piece in the puzzle. You'll find fewer children, more birth control, and less breastfeeding in the West, as opposed to more children, less birth control, and more breastfeeding in Asian cultures. Some even wonder about the effect of more physical activity on cancer risk in Asian women versus sedentary Western women.

Studies on dietary fat and breast cancer have not been able to prove absolutely that high-fat diets are linked to a greater breast cancer risk, however. The fat and breast-cancer issue has polarized breast-cancer researchers. Some will tell you that the proof is in the geography: countries with high-fat diets simply have more breast cancer. Others will tell you that there are too many variables geographically and culturally that need to be studied before the fat theory becomes fact.

What you've probably heard most about is the U.S. Nurses' Health Study, where half of the nurses enrolled (who were followed over several years) received 44 per cent of their daily calories from fat, while the other half received 23 per cent of their daily calories from fat. This study was analyzed by Harvard University's Walter Willett, who concluded that the study showed no difference in breast-cancer risk between the two groups. Similar studies on dietary fat found the same results.

Critics of the Nurses' Health Study argue that, in order to see a difference, the "fat-cutting nurses" should have been getting no more than 15 per cent of their calories from fat. Other problems with dietary fat studies are that the food-frequency questionnaires used to measure what people are eating are pretty crude measurement tools. Researchers also question the timing of dietary fat in a woman's life cycle. Some wonder whether low-fat diets have greater impact on breast-cancer risk in childhood and adolescence, when breasts are still forming, than in adulthood, when breasts are mature.

We may know the answers to some of these questions in 2010, when the results from the largest dietary-fat study to date are due. The Women's Health Initiative is a $628-million health trial involving 164,000 American women. It intends to test whether a low-fat diet that's high in fruits, vegetables, and grains leads to lower breast-cancer incidence in postmenopausal women than the typical Western diet

Finally, researchers published a 1998 report that suggested a 40 per cent increased risk of breast cancer in women who consumed higher levels of trans fatty acids (see Chapters 4 and 8). The risk was highest among women who consume low levels of polyunsaturated fats and high levels of trans fatty acids.

Food, Body Fat, and Environmental Toxins: What We Can't Prove but Suspect

Some environmental scientists, such as Dr. Sandra Steingraber, author of *Living Downstream: An Ecologist Looks at Cancer and the Environment*, hypothesize that body fat serves as an excellent host for fat-soluble toxins, such as certain manmade chemicals known as organochlorines. These substances break down into an estrogenic by-product that may be influencing the increase in certain estrogenic cancers. This is one reason why many cancer activists feel more research is needed about toxic substances and cancer risk. Based on the existing science, we can only say that we suspect, but can't prove, environmental links to cancer. Based on the Ontario task force report on primary cancer prevention, here's what is known.

The most serious hazards affecting our food are what are called persistent toxic substances. These are so named because they are, well, persistent. They remain in the biophysical environment for long periods of time and become widely dispersed, establishing themselves in the plants and animals (including humans!) that ingest them as part of the food chain. Sadly, the ecosystem is incapable of breaking down many of these substances; because they are not naturally occurring chemicals (with their own built-in metabolic pathways for detoxifying themselves), the ecosystem has no way to absorb them. In fact, many of these chemicals have been developed because they are not readily metabolized and detoxified! They stick around and cause any number of adverse health effects, including cancer in humans and animals.

Studies conducted on animals show a positive correlation between organochlorines and breast cancer. A possible link also exists between breast cancer and exposure to xeno-estrogens, estrogenlike substances released into the environment as pesticides or industrial chemicals, which accumulate in body fat. The more estrogen women are exposed to in their lifetimes, the greater their risk of breast cancer. However, evidence of the association between organochlorines (often made up of xeno-estrogens) and breast cancer is inconclusive. Most human populations also now carry detectable levels of suspected carcinogens (e.g., DDT, PCBs) in their body fat, which is why leaner physiques are encouraged (less fat, less toxins).

For more information on environmental causes of cancer, consult my book *Stopping Cancer at the Source*.

DIETARY GUIDELINES FOR PREVENTING CANCER

1. Reduce intake of saturated fats (see Chapters 1, 4, 5, and 8), which is linked to higher rates of colon, ovarian, and prostate cancers. (Red meat is associated more with colon and advanced prostate cancers.)
2. Eat fresh fruits and vegetables daily. They may reduce the risks of a number of cancers, including those of the mouth, pharynx, esophagus, stomach, colon, rectum, larynx, lung, breast, and bladder.
3. Both soluble and insoluble fiber (see Chapter 8) is good for you; experts are not entirely sure why. Is it the vitamins in high-fiber foods? Is it the regularity that fiber promotes? Right now, since all the nutrient-rich foods are also high in fiber, we are promoting high-fiber diets, but some experts think it's better to promote a high fruit and vegetable diet.

The World Cancer Research Fund report specifically recommends the following cancer prevention diet:

- Maintain a normal body weight (with a BMI ranging from 21 to 23. See Chapter 1).
- Moderate daily exercise protects against colon, breast, and lung cancers. Spend an hour daily taking a brisk walk, or an hour weekly of vigorous activity.

- Consume roughly 500 grams of a combination of fruits and vegetables daily (that's five or more portions – see Chapter 4).
- Consume 600 to 800 grams, or more than seven portions, of grains, legumes, roots, or tubers daily (Chapter 4).
- Limit alcohol to two drinks per day for men (or 5 per cent of calories daily); one daily drink for women (or 2.5 per cent of calories daily). This advice works well with the advice in Chapter 6.
- If you must eat red meat, consume no more than 80 grams, or 3 ounces, daily.
- A diet ranging from 15 to 30 per cent of calories from total fat daily is recommended by most panel members of the World Cancer Research Fund report, with a noted objection from Dr. Walter Willett. Willett points out that the studies linking fat and cancer are not well designed to give us enough information. Studies are usually based on total fat intake, not on separating out saturated fat from various animals, trans fatty acids, and unsaturated fats. Based on what we know so far, Willett believes the 15 to 30 per cent fat recommendation is too restrictive, and argues that obesity is also caused by overconsumption of any calorie, not just fat. He recommends that, when saturated fats are replaced by unsaturated fats, there is no evidence of a link between fat and cancer. This is obviously an area in debate. See Chapter 8 for more on this.
- Limit salt consumption to about 6 grams per day. This is consistent with advice on hypertension.
- Limit consumption of refined carbs and sugars (see Chapter 4).

MAKING THE RIGHT CHANGES TO YOUR DIET

What you need to understand about good versus bad diets is that people who consume less saturated fats and fewer empty calories (high-starch or high-sugar items) and more fiber are generally healthier. A low-fat, high-fiber diet will definitely reduce your risk of colon cancer, possibly other cancers, and will definitely reduce your risk of heart disease and diabetes.

THE PROBLEM OF POVERTY

Poverty is an enormous barrier to a healthy diet and lifestyle, and while the problem used to be rampant particularly in the seniors community, it is now more of a problem in families led by single mothers.

Because they may not have the money to spend on transportation, many low-income families shop for food at small convenience stores, where the quality and selection of healthy food products such as fresh vegetables is limited. Ironically, convenience-store prices are generally higher than those at suburban grocery stores. Transportation barriers also exist for the disabled, which again, limit grocery-shopping locations. And since poverty and poor literacy skills often go hand in hand, complicated nutrition labels can be a real barrier to accessing healthy foods.

If you're struggling to put nutritious food on the table, there are things you can do to help put those into your local grocery store:

- Together with others in your community who share the same problem, look into alternative methods of shopping or eating through community kitchens, food-buying clubs, and networking with farms that may be willing to do "field-to-table programs." You could also start a community garden.
- Contact food manufacturers and encourage them to donate all unused fresh produce and other healthy foods to food banks or community kitchens.
- If you're a parent, get your school board to institute a school breakfast and/or lunch program to help children in need eat more nutritiously.
- Contact your city planning department and let them know that your community is in need of good food stores rather than convenience stores.

- In economically strapped communities, it might be worthwhile to contact some of the larger food stores with good selections and encourage them to invest in your community by buying out some of the deadwood retailers (such as pawnshops or money marts) and open some new stores. This trend is seen in many large urban centers as part of urban-renewal programs.

MARKETING BOARD AND PRODUCER ASSOCIATIONS

Provincial and state marketing boards and producer associations are an important part of the food production and distribution system, which work with our farmers. Most of these boards and associations are involved in the quality production of fruits, vegetables, and grains. In the last few years, in response to consumer demand for lower-fat products, the meat and dairy industries, in particular, are making lower-fat products available. There are also a variety of soy manufacturers who are delivering meat and dairy substitutes in the form of tofu burgers, tofu cheeses, or even tofu turkeys.

Understanding grading of meat is another problem. In Canada, consumers believe that the highest-quality grades (AAA) are the healthiest when, in fact, they are often the most fat. To meet AAA criteria, meat has to contain greater marbling (visible fat). Beef with no visible fat is graded B, but it may be leaner. "High-quality" beef must therefore revert to its previous status as a high-fat-containing food that could prove harmful to the consumer's health. So when shopping for meat, be sure to check with your local meat-marketing board to learn what your meat grading refers to.

AVOID RUINING THE RIGHT FOODS

The American Institute for Cancer Research's Diet and Cancer Project, Food Nutrition and the Prevention of Cancer, recommends that by avoiding the following, you'll decrease your risk of cancer:

- Avoid salted foods and table salt whenever possible; season your foods with herbs.
- Avoid eating food that was "left out" for long periods of time; the food can become contaminated with bacteria.
- Avoid eating perishable foods that were not refrigerated.
- Avoid unlabeled foods when travelling in undeveloped or developing countries, as contaminants, additives, and other residues are not properly regulated in these areas.
- Avoid charred food, or meat and fish cooked over an open flame.
- Avoid cured or smoked meats. The nitrites these foods contain are carcinogenic.

THE SKINNY

Cancer cannot be isolated to a single cause, or even to a single food group. But the links between food, nutrition, and cancer are strong enough for recommendations to be made about a "cancer-prevention diet."

Key factors determining whether people develop cancer are environmental. Diets higher in plant-based foods and lower in saturated fats are the basis for preventing or protecting against certain cancers. Cancer is indeed multifactorial, as the discussion on risk co-factors at the beginning of this chapter emphasizes. Insufficient activity is one of the most important co-factors in diet and cancer risks. The World Cancer Research Fund report estimates that 30 to 40 per cent of cancer incidence would drop if people ate a healthy, balanced diet (see Chapter 8 and earlier) and were more active. That accounts for 3 to 4 million cases of cancer per year.

Overall, we know from a myriad of good studies that lowering our fat intake and increasing more nutrient-rich grains and vegetables (which also increases our fiber) is considered to lower the risk of certain cancers. Also, lowering body fat appears to lower the risk of accumulating fat-soluble toxins, which could be linked to certain cancers. In the following chapters, you'll learn about various approaches to lowering dietary and body fat.

CHAPTER 4

A Good Look at Low-Fat Diets

Adiet is considered "low fat" when it restricts calories from fat to below 30 per cent daily. There are dozens of established low-fat diets on the market, but they vary from extremely low-fat diets to more moderate low-fat diets. All low-fat diets are modeled after the "originators" of the very low-fat diet as we know it today – Nathan Pritikin, who popularized low-fat eating in the 1950s, and Dean Ornish, who reframed the original Pritikin diet in the late 1970s. This chapter discusses these two diets in detail, since they remain the most well-known and most effective diets for people who are extremely obese and at high risk for dying from an obesity-related health problem. I've coined the terms *Ornish-styled* and *Pritikin-styled* to mean any diet using the general principles of very low-fat eating.

The short answer to the question "Do low-fat diets work?" is yes. The short answer to "Do low-fat diets usually fail?" is yes. The main discussion about low-fat diets centers on why – in both cases – they work *and* fail. And how can you, as a consumer, understand where you fit in the low-fat puzzle. This chapter explores the science-based evidence of very low-fat diets, which restrict calories from fat to about 10 per cent of daily intake.

Although there are a range of low-fat diets far more generous in fat calories (from 15 to 25 per cent), to understand low-fat diets it's crucial to understand the history of the very low-fat diet's development and what it was designed to do. It also examines the controversy about low-fat diets, and the arguments its critics have made with respect to failure.

DEFINING LOW-FAT DIETS

A low-fat diet should really be described as "how to reverse heart disease without drugs." These diets recommend low-fat options whenever possible and emphasize complex carbohydrates such as whole-grain breads, rice, and pasta; high-fiber vegetables, fruits, and beans; and high-fiber oats and cereals. The average calorie intake for people on a very low-fat diet is about 1,200 to 1,500 calories a day, with no more than 10 per cent of daily calories coming from either saturated or unsaturated fat. Moderate exercise is recommended along with the diets.

Low-fat diets are not rocket science: eating fewer calories and exercising will always lead to weight loss. Since there are nine calories to each gram of fat, eliminating fat from the diet is the shortest route to consuming fewer calories. Protein and carbohydrates have only four calories per gram. So eating less fat, in theory, allows you to eat more food and remain more satiated. Restricting the saturated fat, which is the fat that raises our "bad cholesterol" – the LDL, or low-density lipoproteins – will lower our cholesterol levels, a key component for people who are candidates for this diet.

There are two groups of people who can benefit from a low-fat diet. The first group comprises those who need to lose weight because they are in very poor health and are "heart attacks waiting to happen." In this case, they might have soaring cholesterol or high blood pressure (both discussed later), evidence of cardiovascular disease, a history of past heart attacks or angina or even stroke. The other group are those who are obese, or those who are *very serious* about losing weight to optimize their health and sense of well being but who have not yet developed an obesity-related disease. People in the second group are worried about developing an obesity-related disease; they've seen family members and friends fall prey to these diseases and fear they are next. They love their families; they are ready, motivated, and may even have the Type A personality of being obsessive and perfectionists in other areas of their lives. Once committed to a project, they may live by the motto "Failure is not an option."

But most people who want to lose weight fall into a third group: those of us who want to look better and feel better about our bodies but who are not in poor health otherwise. Our motivations are image and self-esteem. For this group, a low-fat diet is likely going to fail, because it is very difficult to stick to in daily life. It is so difficult, in fact, that threats of dire health consequences and/or loss of life are usually required in order to keep people on a low-fat diet. It has to be almost a "religion."

Low-fat diets are optimally designed for people who need to reverse heart disease, frequently a complication of poorly controlled type 2 diabetes. People with advanced heart disease can eliminate their need for surgery by following these fat-restricted diets. Researchers have studied low-fat diets since the 1950s, when Nathan Pritikin, the pioneer of the low-fat diet, first preached its virtues. Iron-clad scientific evidence supports that the longer people stay on a low-fat diet, the more their heart disease improves. When cardiologists or endocrinologists (who manage diabetes) see morbidly obese patients whom they estimate will be dead within a year from a heart attack, they may put them on a Pritikin Diet – the most extreme of the low-fat diets, which restricts daily calories from fat to no more than 7 per cent of calories per day. Medical advice is blunt: "If you want to live another year, go on this diet today." Those that do, and stay on it, lose the weight they need to lose, lower their cholesterol, and can *dramatically* lower their risk of death from obesity-related diseases. No one disputes that a low-fat diet works for these people. Low-fat diets are not designed as "weight loss" diets but as diets that can reverse obesity-related diseases or, in clinicalspeak, "morbidity."

THE PRITIKIN DIET

In the late 1950s Nathan Pritikin was himself diagnosed with heart disease. Pritikin developed a low-fat, high-fiber diet and also began a moderate exercise program. He successfully reversed his heart disease, and developed the Pritikin Diet based on his own experience. All nutrition experts as well as heart-disease experts praise this diet for its safety and reliability, though critics of the diet point out that it is difficult to follow. The Pritikin Diet is mostly vegetarian, encouraging you to rely on whole grains and vegetables for most of your meals. It allows less than 10 per cent of daily calories from fat, or approximately 7 per cent. This diet ensures that you're getting fiber, but very little cholesterol and saturated fat. Most people are encouraged to eat frequently during the day to keep their blood sugar stable. It discourages processed foods and animal protein, and also requires you to exercise daily by simply walking forty-five minutes each day. (As discussed in Chapter 3, a low-fat diet will also help to prevent colon cancer; the benefits of preventing other cancers are unclear.)

By following the Pritikin Diet, you'll average about 400 calories a meal, because you'll be eating foods that average about 4 calories per gram, instead of the 9 calories per gram that fat provides. Meals will include a maximum of about 3.5 ounces of animal protein per day, two servings of fat-free dairy food a day, and a range of unprocessed foods such as fruits, vegetables, and complex grains and carbohydrates. In light of more information on good fats, the Pritikin Diet has been revised to encourage that the fat one consumes during the day be a "good fat."

Most sensible weight-loss diets, government guidelines on meal planning, and diabetes associations throughout the world loosely model meal planning on this diet, but allow for far-more-generous portions of protein and fat (see Chapter 8). What is key to remember about the Pritikin Diet is that it is not intended as a weight-loss diet; it is a lifesaving measure to reverse heart disease or factors that can predispose you to a heart attack. Weight loss is the "fringe benefit" of a Pritikin Diet.

THE ORNISH DIET

Another "low-fat pioneer" is Dr. Dean Ornish, whose own program, developed in the early 1970s, borrows heavily from the Pritikin Diet, with these differences:

- You're allowed up to 10 per cent of daily calories from fat, and advised to have three grams of "good" fats each day, what Ornish insists is an ample daily quantity.
- Exercise is necessary, as in the Pritikin Diet, but Ornish encourages spiritual exercise too, in the form of meditation and stress reduction. On the Ornish program, the diet alone is not enough to achieve his dramatic results of heart-disease reversal; the daily exercise and stress reduction is crucial.

There is undisputed research that demonstrates the value of lifestyle changes, not just dietary changes, in reversing heart disease. Ornish states that his research shows that, in patients who followed his entire program (not just the diet), angina decreased by 91 per cent and their cholesterol levels fell by 40 per cent without the use of medications. The simple fact is that most people can avoid heart surgery by following a low-fat diet program correctly.

Meals on a Low-Fat Diet

To get a good idea of what a low-fat diet looks like, here is a typical sample menu for the day. Breakfast might consist of one glass of freshly squeezed orange juice or a fresh orange; a large bowl of a plain cold cereal (such as Bran Flakes or Cheerios) with fat-free milk, or a large bowl of hot cereal with low-fat milk (sweeteners can be used instead of sugar); one or two pieces of toast with preserves or a fat-free cheese or spread of some sort; coffee or tea (black or with fat-free milk).

Lunch might consist of a large sandwich with lean meat (turkey, chicken, tuna, etc.) on whole-wheat bread, with a large salad (dressing could include a "good fat," such as olive oil – see Chapter 6), and a low-fat yogurt.

Dinner might consist of four ounces of lean chicken or fish, with two medium potatoes, two different, interesting vegetables prepared in various ways (such as steamed spinach, bok choy, green beans, or broccoli, and grilled eggplant or baked spaghetti squash). A green and a colored vegetable with dinner adds variety for the palate. Dessert could be chopped fruit with a low-fat ice cream, yogurt, or other fat-free topping.

Snacks during the day can include bean dips such as hummus or refried beans with a whole-grain bread or pita; fruits; baby carrots; low-fat yogurts or cheeses; or whole-grain-based snacks and cereals.

As you can see, this is a healthy, varied diet for one day. There are hundreds of things you can eat on a low-fat diet, and following a diet such as this should not leave you feeling hungry. The weight loss to expect is about 1.5 to 2 pounds, per week, which is a healthy, sustainable weight loss.

WHY LOW-FAT DIETS FAIL

By the mid-1980s, nutrition and medical experts began to publish the amazing results of heart-disease reversal in people who were on the Pritikin or Ornish programs. Low-fat dieting was suddenly the "answer" to health and longevity, and people who were not obese and who did not have signs of heart disease flocked to this very low-fat diet – a diet never intended for them. Indeed, these diets are far too restrictive as weight-loss programs for the masses. The media, too, largely misunderstood the original intent of the Pritikin and Ornish diets. People began to think that a "low-fat diet" meant that, so long as products did not contain fat (saturated or unsaturated), they could eat all they wanted and they'd lose weight. In short, to say that "low-fat diets fail" is a bit like saying, "I got pregnant because I forgot to take my birth-control pill."

Then there was the problem with diet failure in people who did follow the Pritikin or Ornish programs. In these cases, people didn't understand how to "use" the diets; many of them lacked enough knowledge about food preparation and food variety to vary their diet with enough interesting foods to balance the loss of fat-based foods. (Buying good food and preparing it well, after all, demands some knowledge of food and nutrition.) People that don't live in large urban centers don't have access to the variety of foods, because their local grocery stores may not carry any vegetables other than run-of-the-mill salad fixings and broccoli, carrots, etc. The result is that many people were hungry and bored with their food.

So people on low-fat diets began to fill up on simple carbohydrates, such as sugar, white flour, and white rice, which gets absorbed too quickly by the body and causes blood sugar to increase, triggering the body to pump out insulin to "clean up" the sugar in the blood. Insulin also increases appetite, and too much insulin accelerates the conversion of calories into body fat. Insulin not only keeps blood sugar in check, it also keeps the levels of "good" cholesterol (HDL – high-density lipoproteins), "bad" cholesterol (LDL – low-density lipoproteins), and triglycerides in check.

People who load up on simple carbohydrates can eventually develop insulin resistance, in which the body is not making enough insulin or the body isn't using insulin efficiently; in this case, your LDL levels and your triglycerides rise, but, more important, your HDL levels fall, which can lead to heart disease. When insulin and blood-sugar levels are in control, cholesterol levels will return to normal, which will cut your risk of heart disease and stroke. People who have insulin resistance will be diagnosed with type 2 diabetes. (Diets that are best for people with type 2 diabetes are those designed with a diabetes educator, which will meet your individual needs. This is discussed in Chapter 8.)

Meanwhile, the food industry had responded to public interest in "low fat" by creating foods with deceptive labels, encouraging "low-fat snacking."

Clearly, filling up on simple carbohydrates is not what the low-fat diet "designers" such as Pritikin or Ornish intended or ever encouraged; if you follow their diet, by eating complex carbohydrates such as unrefined whole-wheat bread, brown rice, fruits, vegetables, and beans, you will get more fiber, which slows the digestion and conversion of these carbohydrates into glucose, thus preventing a sudden spike in your blood sugar and the consequent spike in insulin output.

In essence, the main philosophy and intent of very low-fat diets such as Pritikin's and Ornish's is upheld by the top nutritionists: eating lots of plant-based foods is best, and a low-fat diet does reverse heart disease without the need for surgery or medication. It's been long established, too, that a 5- to 10-per-cent reduction in weight can reverse diabetes, hypertension, and high cholesterol. Thus, the claims of a low-fat diet are accurate. However, simply eliminating fat and eating all the "low-fat" products you want is a gross misinterpretation of low-fat eating.

THE IMPACT OF "LOW-FAT" PRODUCTS

As mentioned, since the late 1970s, North Americans have been deluged with low-fat products. In 1990, the U.S. government launched Healthy People 2000, a campaign to urge manufacturers to double their output of low-fat products by the year 2000. Since 1990, more than a thousand new fat-free or low-fat products have been introduced into North American supermarkets annually.

Most of these low-fat products, however, actually encourage us to eat more. For example, if a bag of regular chips has nine grams of fat per serving (one serving usually equals about five chips, or one handful), you will more likely stick to that one handful. However, if you find a low-fat brand of chips that boasts "50 per cent less fat" per serving, you're more likely to eat the whole bag (feeling good about eating "low-fat" chips), which can easily triple your fat intake.

Low-fat or fat-free foods work by tricking our bodies with ingredients that mimic the functions of fat in foods. This is often achieved by using modified fats that are only partially metabolized – if metabolized at all. While some foods reduce the fat by actually removing the fat (skim milk, lean cuts of meat), most low-fat foods employ a variety of "fat copycats" to preserve the taste and texture of the food. Water, for example, is often combined with carbohydrates and protein to mimic a particular texture or taste, as is the case with a variety of baked goods or cake mixes. In general, though, the low-fat "copycats" are carbohydrate-based, protein-based, or even fat-based.

Carbohydrate-based ingredients are starches and gums that are often used as thickening agents to create the texture of fat. You'll find these in abundance in sauces, gravies, frozen desserts, baked goods, and low-fat salad dressings (which are considered off-limits by many nutritionists because they interfere with phytochemicals, discussed in Chapter 8). These run between zero and four calories per gram. Protein-based low-fat ingredients are created by processing proteins to make them behave differently. For example, by taking proteins such as whey or egg white, and heating or blending them at high speeds, you can create the look and feel of a "creamy" dish. Soy and corn proteins are often used in these cases. You'll find these ingredients in low-fat cheese, butter, mayonnaise, salad dressings, frozen dairy desserts, sour cream, and baked goods. These foods run between one to four calories per gram.

Low-fat foods that use fat-based ingredients tailor the fat so that we do not absorb or metabolize it fully. These ingredients are found in chocolate, chocolate coatings, margarine, spreads, sour cream, and cheese. You can also use these ingredients as low-fat substitutes for frying foods (you do this when you fry eggs in margarine, for example). Olestra, the fat substitute found in abundance in the United States (but not approved for use in Canada), is an example of a fat substitute that is not absorbed by our bodies, and so provides no calories. Caprenin and salatrim are examples of partially absorbed fats (they contain more long-chain fatty acids), and are the more traditional fat-based low-fat ingredients. These are roughly five calories per gram.

There's no question that low-fat foods are designed to give you more freedom of choice with a low-fat diet, which supposedly allows you to cut your fat without compromising taste. Studies show that taste outperforms "nutrition" in your brain. Yet these products paradoxically helped to create the obesity epidemic discussed in Chapter 1 by encouraging us to eat more calories, even though we are reducing our overall fat intake.

What remains true is that low-fat or fat-free products are, in fact, *lower in fat* and when used in moderation can substitute for the "bad foods" you know you shouldn't have but cannot live without. If you simply treat a low-fat product like its high-fat original, the product can work for you. But if you double the amount because it's "low fat," it will work against you.

CONFUSING LABELING

Confusing labeling contributes to the problem of selecting a truly low-fat product. In Canada, ingredients on labels are listed according to weight, with the "most" listed first. If sugar is the first ingredient, you know the product contains mostly sugar. The lower sugar is on the list, the less sugar in the product. The nutrition information on the label should also list the total amount of carbohydrates in a serving of the food. That amount includes both natural and added sugars.

Whenever a product says it is "calorie-reduced" or "carbohydrate-reduced," it means it has 50 per cent fewer calories or carbohydrates compared to the original product. But something that was originally 7,000 calories isn't much better at 3,500. You still have to limit your intake.

The label "cholesterol-free" or "low cholesterol" means that the product doesn't have any, or much, animal fat (hence, cholesterol). This doesn't mean "low fat." Pure vegetable oil doesn't come from animals but is still pure fat! What is highly misunderstood about cholesterol, however, is that what is important is not the cholesterol in the product, but the type of fat in the product, which will raise your cholesterol. An example of terrible cholesterol confusion can be found in the consumer outcry over the low-fat margarines of the 1980s and 1990s. Low-cholesterol or fat-free margarines were developed as alternatives to butter and saturated fat. But the hydrolysis process involved in making a liquid unsaturated fat solid created trans fatty acids, which raised cholesterol levels and were metabolized by the body as saturated fat. Fat labeling is discussed more in Chapter 8, but the confusion over margarines prevail. Margarines with less than 60 to 80 per cent oil (9 to 11 grams of fat) will contain 1 to 3 grams of trans fatty acids per serving, compared to butter, which is 53 per cent saturated fat. Trans fatty acids (a.k.a. trans fats) are not mentioned on labels; rather, the trans fat is labeled as part of the total fat. This adds to cholesterol confusion. Consumer groups point out that it is unethical for foods with two grams or less trans fats per serving not to list their trans fats on the label when foods with as little as half a gram of saturated fat have it listed.

Remember too, a label that screams Low Fat means that the product has less than three grams of fat *per serving*. In potato-chip country, that means about six potato chips. (I don't know anybody who ever ate one serving of potato chips!) So if you eat the whole bag of "low-fat" chips, you're still eating a lot of fat. Even the labels on fat-free cooking sprays are misleading. Cooking sprays that say they are for fat-free cooking still add fat unless you spray for less than one second (which delivers seven calories).

Products that are "light" (or "lite") mean that there is 25 to 50 per cent less of some ingredient in that product. It could be fat, cholesterol, salt, or sugar, or less food coloring, and therefore the designation is frequently misleading.

"Sugar-free" in the language of labels simply means sucrose-free. That doesn't mean the product is carbohydrate-free, as in: dextrose-free, lactose-free, glucose-free, or fructose-free. Check the labels for all things ending in "ose" to find out the sugar content; you're not just looking for sucrose. Watch out for "no added sugar," "without added sugar," or "no sugar added." This means: "We didn't put the sugar in, God did." Again, reading the number of carbohydrates on the nutrition information label is the most accurate way to know the amount of sugar in the product. Nutrition claims in big, bold statements can be misleading.

Shuffling off to Buffalo or Seattle for a shopping trip? American labels that read "sugar-free" contain less than 0.5 grams of sugars per serving, while a "reduced-sugar" food contains at least 25 per cent less sugar per serving than the regular product. If the label also states that the product is not a reduced- or low-calorie food, or it is not for weight control, it's got enough sugar in there to make you think twice.

Serving sizes in the United States are also listed differently. Foods that are similar are given the same type of serving size defined by the U.S. Food and Drug Administration (FDA). That means that five cereals that all weigh X grams per cup will share the same serving sizes.

Calories (how much energy) and calories from fat (how much fat) are also listed per serving of food in the United States. Total carbohydrate, dietary fiber, sugars, other carbohydrates (which means starches), total fat, saturated fat, cholesterol, sodium, potassium, and vitamin and minerals are given in Percent Daily Values, based on the 2,000-calorie diet recommended by the U.S. government. (In Canada, Recommended Nutrient Intake [RNI] is used for vitamins and minerals.)

UNREAL WEIGHT-LOSS EXPECTATIONS

Many people report that a low-fat diet failed because they did not lose as much weight as they had hoped, or weight loss came too slowly. Any diet that advertises dramatic weight loss in a short period of time is suspect; diets that starve the body of nutrients will also make the body more efficient at gaining weight, which is why so many dieters will cycle and yo-yo as they go from radical diets to normal eating.

Many people who expected weight loss solely from the diet, without incorporating moderate exercise, are also disappointed. No diet, unless it's starvation-based, will work optimally without activity.

Aging naturally slows our metabolism too. Women, in particular, find that, as they approach their late thirties, they can put on weight even when they have not changed their eating patterns.

The impact of stress and emotional health should be noted. People tend to crave simple carbohydrates while under stress. Cortisol, which is a stress hormone we make, can also increase appetites. On the flip side, when people are depressed, they tend to lose interest in food and will lose weight more rapidly (although others gain).

There may be other health conditions that are interfering with weight loss, such as hypothyroidism, commonly diagnosed in women particularly. Several medications can cause weight gain or bloat as well. Generally, before undertaking a low-fat diet, be sure that you know the status of your current health and what factors may be aggravating your efforts.

WHAT THE CRITICS SAY ABOUT LOW-FAT DIETS

When a very low-fat diet is understood in its proper context, there is little to criticize. People can dramatically improve their health and reverse heart disease on a very low-fat diet. However, when one takes this diet *out of context* and applies it to the general population as a "weight-loss diet" it can be harshly criticized. Ninety-nine per cent of the criticism surrounding low-fat diets stems from a misunderstanding of what a Pritikin-type or Ornish-type diet was designed to do: *prevent or reverse heart disease without drugs or surgery*. If you don't have heart disease, and are not currently at risk for it, you should not be on a diet this restrictive in fat. Period. People with type 2 diabetes should not go on this diet without attending a diabetes education course, consulting with a certified diabetes educator (CDE), and planning a diabetes meal plan with a CDE. Usually the proper diet for someone with type 2 diabetes must incorporate more protein and fat. Reasonable healthy diets for the average person, as well as diabetes diets, are discussed in Chapter 8.

That said, the valid criticism surrounding low-fat diets is that newer research since the development of these diets has shown that fat is not equal; there are good and bad fats, as discussed in Chapter 8. So low-fat diets that restrict calories from fat to extremes (such as Pritikin's at less than 10, or about 7 per cent, or Ornish's at a maximum of 10 per cent) can deprive people of the undisputed benefits of good fats, which are shown to raise HDL, or "good cholesterol," and protect us from many diseases; they are also proven to be necessary in order for the various phytochemicals from plants to work in the body. The latest Pritikin and Ornish diet information recognizes the benefits of good fats, but advises that, within the limits, one can satisfy the good-fat daily requirements by taking three grams of fish oil or flaxseed oil per day. Critics argue that many important nutrients we derive from vegetables are fat-soluble; therefore, a diet too restricted in fat deprives us of these nutrients, notably vitamins A, D, E, and K.

Critics also point out that there may be flaws in Ornish's research and his published success rates. For example, in his program, the very low-fat diet is recommended along with an exercise regime that includes meditation. Thus, it is difficult, critics say, truly to measure whether the dramatic health benefits he boasts are solely due to the diet or whether the lifestyle measures accompanying the diet are the real reason for the success. In other words, if people followed a less restrictive diet such as the 40-30-30 program (40 per cent carbs; 30 per cent protein; 30 per cent fat) discussed in Chapter 8, and exercised and meditated too, would they see the same results?

Many nutritionists feel that heart health can be achieved with much more good fat, as well as exercise. The Mediterranean diet in Chapter 6 has been shown in some studies to reverse heart disease too, without going to the extremes of Pritikin and Ornish; the calorie-per-day intake is still about the same – 1,500 (or more for larger builds).

A final and central criticism of very low-fat diets is that they are hard to stick to, a fact that remains even when the diet is viewed within its proper context – as a heart-disease-reversal diet. Very low-fat diets ought to include an education component for all people beginning the diet, just as diabetes meal planning does; sometimes a low-fat diet candidate is educated, but it varies with the health-care practitioner. Studies show that, when there is an education component to a low-fat diet, which teaches people about healthy eating, innovative ways to prepare low-fat recipes, where to shop, and types of activities that can count as "exercise," people can stay on the program and feel good. People tend to view exercise, for example, as a task within a gym, rather than as a life activity, such as gardening, forty-five-minute walks that incorporate errands and shopping, or just going to the zoo or an art museum.

BEST CANDIDATES FOR LOW-FAT DIETS

The best candidates for low-fat diets are non-smokers at risk of dying from a heart attack or stroke (more broadly known as cardiovascular disease, which is one of the most common complications of obesity). If you smoke, and think a low-fat diet will improve your health, you're under a delusion. In this case, make every effort to quit smoking first before you go on a low-fat diet. Doing both at the same time is very difficult, although not impossible. Being on a low-fat diet and continuing to smoke does you no good from a cardiovascular point of view. If you had to pick one, quitting smoking will dramatically decrease your risk of dying from a heart attack or stroke. The non-smoking population most at risk of dying from a heart attack or stroke have one or more of the following conditions:

HIGH CHOLESTEROL

Cholesterol is a whitish, waxy fat made in vast quantities by the liver. It is also known as a lipid, the umbrella name for the many different fats found in the body. That's why liver or other organ meats are high in cholesterol! Cholesterol is needed to make hormones as well as cell membranes. Dietary cholesterol is found only in foods from animals and fish. The daily maximum amount of dietary cholesterol recommended by Health Canada is 300 mg. If you have high cholesterol, the excess cholesterol in your blood can lead to narrowed arteries, which can lead to a heart attack. Saturated fat, discussed in detail later, is often a culprit when it comes to high cholesterol, which is why a low-fat diet is useful.

But the highest levels of cholesterol are due to a genetic defect in the liver; low-fat diets are useful to keep this condition in check.

In Canada, total blood cholesterol levels are measured in millimoles per liter (mmol/L). If you're older than thirty, cholesterol levels of less than 5.2 mmol/L are considered healthy. If your doctor tells you that your cholesterol levels are between 5.2 and 6.2 mmol/L, discuss lifestyle changes that can lower cholesterol levels. If your levels are greater than 6.2 mmol/L, and your lifestyle changes were not successful, your doctor may recommend cholesterol-lowering drugs.

For people eighteen to twenty-nine years of age, a cholesterol level less than 4.7 mmol/L is considered healthy, while a level ranging between 4.7 and 5.7 mmol/L is considered too high, warranting some lifestyle/dietary changes. In this age group, a reading greater than 5.7 may even warrant cholesterol-lowering drugs. High cholesterol is also called hypercholesterolemia. Another term used in conjunction with high cholesterol is hyperlipidemia, which refers to an elevation of lipids (fats) in the bloodstream; lipids include cholesterol and triglycerides (the most common form of fat from food sources in our bodies). For adults, a triglyceride level less than 2.3 mmol/L is considered healthy.

Total blood cholesterol levels are guidelines only. You also have to look at the relative proportion of high-density lipoprotein (HDL), or "good cholesterol," to low-density lipoprotein (LDL) level, or "bad cholesterol," in the blood. If you're older than thirty, an LDL reading of less than 3.4 mmol/L and an HDL reading of more than 0.9 mmol/L is considered healthy; if you're eighteen to twenty-nine, an LDL reading of less than 3.0 mmol/L and an HDL reading of more than 0.9 mmol/L is considered healthy.

CHOLESTEROL-LOWERING DRUGS

For many, losing weight and modifying fat intake simply aren't enough to bring cholesterol levels down to optimal levels. You may be a candidate for one of the numerous cholesterol-lowering drugs that have hit the market in recent years. These medications, when combined with a low-fat, low-cholesterol diet, target the intestine, blocking food absorption, and/or the liver, where they interfere with the processing of cholesterol. These are strong drugs, however, and ought to be a last resort after you have really given a low-fat/low-cholesterol diet a chance. You might be given a combination of cholesterol-lowering medications to try with a low-cholesterol diet. It's important to ask about all side effects accompanying your medication, because they can include gastrointestinal problems, allergic reactions, blood disorders, and depression. There have not been enough studies on women taking these drugs to truly know how they interact with women's particular health conditions.

Table 4.1

Your Cholesterol

The following are the 2001 guidelines recommended by the Canadian Heart and Stroke Foundation for people aged thirty and older:

	GOOD	POOR
Total Cholesterol	below 5.2	above 6.2
LDL Cholesterol	below 3.4	above 3.4
HDL Cholesterol	above 0.9	below 0.9
Triglycerides	below 2.3	above 2.3

HYPERTENSION (A.K.A. HIGH BLOOD PRESSURE)

About 12 per cent of Canadian adults suffer from hypertension, or high blood pressure. What is blood pressure? The blood flows from the heart into the arteries (blood vessels), pressing against the artery walls. Think about a liquid-soap dispenser. When you want soap, you need to pump it out by pressing down on the little dispenser pump, the "heart" of the dispenser. The liquid soap is the "blood" and the little tube through which the soap flows is the "artery." The pressure that's exerted on the wall of the tube is therefore the "blood pressure."

When the tube is hollow and clean, you needn't pump very hard to get the soap; it comes out easily. But when the tubing in your dispenser gets narrower as a result of old, hardened, gunky liquid soap blocking the tube, you have to pump down much harder to get any soap, while the force the soap exerts against the tube is increased. Obviously, this is a simplistic explanation of a very complex problem, but essentially the narrowing of the arteries forces your heart to work harder to pump the blood, causing high blood pressure. If this goes on too long, your heart muscle enlarges and becomes weaker, which can lead to a heart attack. Higher pressure can also weaken the walls of your blood vessels, which can cause a stroke.

The term *hypertension* refers to the tension or force exerted on your artery walls. (Hyper means "too much," as in "too much tension.") Blood pressure is measured in two readings: X over Y. The X is the systolic pressure, which is the pressure that occurs during the heart's contraction. The Y is the diastolic pressure, which is the pressure that occurs when the heart rests between contractions. In "liquid soap" terms, the systolic pressure occurs when you press the pump down; the diastolic pressure occurs when you release your hand from the pump and allow it to rise back to its "resting" position.

In the general population, target blood-pressure readings are less than 130 over 85 (<130/85). Readings greater than 130/85 are considered by diabetes educators to be too high for people with diabetes, but in the general population, readings of 140/90 or higher are generally considered borderline, although for some people this is still considered a normal reading. For the general population, 140/90 is "lecture time," when your doctor will begin to counsel you about dietary and lifestyle habits. By 160/100, many people are prescribed a hypertensive drug, which is designed to lower blood pressure.

Obesity, as we saw in Chapter 1, is the chief cause of hypertension. Hypertension is also exacerbated by tobacco and alcohol consumption, and by too much sodium (salt) in the diet.

If high blood pressure runs in the family, you're considered at greater risk of developing hypertension. High blood pressure can also be caused by kidney disorders (which may be initially caused by diabetes) or pregnancy (known as pregnancy-induced hypertension). Medications are also common culprits. Estrogen-containing medications (such as oral contraceptives), non-steroidal anti-inflammatory drugs (NSAIDs) such as ibuprofen, nasal decongestants, cold remedies, appetite suppressants, certain antidepressants, and other drugs can all increase blood pressure. Be sure to check with your pharmacist. If you can't lower your blood pressure through lifestyle changes such as losing weight and increasing physical activity, you may be a candidate for a blood-pressure-lowering drug.

MORBID OBESITY

Morbid obesity can be reversed with a low-fat diet, but since so many people who are morbidly obese are compulsive overeaters or binge eaters, finding additional support with a therapist or an organization such as Overeaters Anonymous is highly recommended. Before you consider drastic measures such as bariatric surgery (stomach stapling), a low-fat diet is a wise first step.

RECOVERING FROM A HEART ATTACK

A heart attack is clinically known as a myocardial infarction (MI). The myocardium is the clinical name for "heart muscle." An MI occurs when there is not enough, or any, blood supply to the myocardium – something that happens when one of the coronary arteries is blocked. A coronary artery is an artery that supplies blood to the heart muscle. Roughly 90 per cent of heart attacks are due to a blood clot, which is a clog in your blood vessels.

You can recover from a heart attack, but the damage resulting from it greatly depends on how long the blood supply to the heart muscle was cut off. A low-fat diet can prevent another heart attack. In other words, the same diet designed to prevent a first heart attack can also be used to prevent recurrent episodes.

RECOVERING FROM A STROKE

Cardiovascular disease puts you at risk for not just a heart attack but a "brain attack," or stroke, which occurs when a blood clot travels to your brain and stops the flow of blood and oxygen carried to the nerve cells in that area. When that happens, cells may die or vital functions controlled by the brain can be temporarily or permanently damaged. Bleeding or a rupture from the affected blood vessel can lead to a very serious situation, including death. About 80 per cent of strokes are caused by the blockage of an artery in the neck or brain, known as an "ischemic stroke"; the remainder are caused by a burst blood vessel in the brain that causes bleeding into or around the brain.

Since the 1960s, the death rate from strokes has dropped by 50 per cent. This drop is largely due to public-awareness campaigns regarding diet and lifestyle modification (quitting smoking, eating low-fat foods, and exercising), as well as the introduction of blood-pressure-lowering drugs and cholesterol-lowering drugs, which have helped people maintain normal blood pressure and cholesterol levels.

Obesity, inactivity, and, especially, smoking spell ANOTHER STROKE unless you make some lifestyle changes. To repeat, a low-fat diet can help prevent a first stroke, as well as a recurring stroke.

MAKING A LOW-FAT DIET WORK

Once you've consulted with your doctor about beginning a low-fat diet specifically for weight loss (unlike the Pritikin or Ornish programs, designed to prevent or reverse heart disease), the following tips can help make a low-fat diet successful and easier to stay on:

1. Consume one or more of these "power plants" daily – nutritionally packed plant-based foods (listed in alphabetical order):

   - beans (protein-rich, loaded with iron, folic acid, and fiber; best selections: black, kidney, pinto, garbanzo, lentil, or navy)
   - broccoli (rich in vitamin C, carotenoids, and folic acid)
   - cantaloupe (one-quarter is almost equal to a full day's requirement of vitamins A and C)
   - oranges (rich in vitamin C, folic acid, and fiber)
   - spinach and kale (loaded with vitamin C, carotenoids, calcium, and fiber)

- sweet potatoes or yams (amazingly packed with carotenoids, vitamin C, potassium and fiber – substitute for potatoes when you can)
- watermelon (packed with vitamin C and carotenoids).

2. Newer margarines that contain sterol or stanol esters, which are plant extracts that lower cholesterol, are considered to be healthy alternatives to butter and regular margarines with trans fatty acids. These newer margarines are only for people who have high cholesterol. Two or three teaspoons are the daily recommendation. They're not recommended for children. Margarines made with omega oils are also good choices.

3. You can replace many meats quite easily with meatless versions that taste almost the same. Meatless substitutes for burgers, hot dogs, chicken nuggets, and so forth have much lower levels of saturated fat and higher levels of fiber and soy. Even Burger King recently introduced a veggie burger that won accolades from *Nutrition Action* newsletter, so long as the condiments on it are not fattening.

4. When eating Chinese food, use rice to help cut the fat; when eating Italian food, choose thin pastas and red sauces. Pizza calories can be cut by ordering a pizza with half the cheese. The best choices, of course, are vegetarian pizzas, or, instead of red meat, ask for chicken. You can also order a no-cheese pizza. Avoid stuffed crusts and multi-meat pizzas. Order a salad with the pizza, and skip the bread sticks, wings, and all the other high-fat sides.

5. When you eat a lot of carbohydrates, even though they may be touted as "low fat," the calories from the sugar and carbohydrates are stored as fat. The more refined the sugar and flour in the carbohydrate, the faster it converts to glucose and digests, and the faster you get hungry again. To avoid

this scenario, choose carbohydrate foods that have a "low glycemic value." "The Glycemic Index," in the table below, helps you rate carbohydrates by how quickly they convert into glucose. Table 4.3, "How Your Food Breaks Down," helps you determine which foods convert to glucose faster. The longer a food takes to break down into glucose, the less hungry you'll feel, the less you'll eat, and the less fat you'll become!

Table 4.2

The Glycemic Index

The glycemic index (GI) shows the rise in blood sugar from various carbohydrates. Therefore, planning your low-fat diet using the GI can help you prevent the insulin spike that so many low-fat dieters fall prey to. Use more foods with a low GI and less foods with a high GI. In general, foods high in fiber have a lower GI. The glycemic index was developed at the University of Toronto, and measures the rate at which various foods convert to glucose, which is assigned a value of 100. Higher numbers indicate a more rapid absorption of glucose. The following list is a sample only. This is not an index of food energy values or calories; some low-GI foods are high in fat, while some high-GI foods are low in fat. Keep in mind that these values differ depending upon what else you're eating with that food and how the food is prepared.

SAMPLE G.I. FOOD VALUES

Sugars

Glucose = 100

Honey = 87

Table sugar = 59

Fructose = 20

Snacks

Mars Bar = 68

Potato chips = 51

Sponge cake = 46

Fish sticks = 38

Tomato soup = 38

Sausages = 28

Peanuts = 13

SAMPLE G.I. FOOD VALUES

Cereals
Corn Flakes = 80
Shredded Wheat = 67
Muesli = 66
All-Bran = 51
Oatmeal = 49

Breads
White = 69
Buckwheat = 51

Fruits
Raisins = 64
Banana = 62
Orange juice = 46
Orange = 40
Apple = 39

Dairy Products
Ice cream = 36
Yogurt = 36
Milk = 34
Skim milk = 32

Root Vegetables
Parsnips = 97
Carrots = 92
Instant mashed potatoes = 80
New boiled potato = 70
Beets = 64
Yam = 51
Sweet potato = 48

Pasta and Rice
White rice = 72
Brown rice = 66
Spaghetti (white) = 50
Spaghetti (whole wheat)= 42

Legumes
Frozen peas = 51
Baked beans = 40
Chickpeas = 36
Lima beans = 36
Butter beans = 36
Black-eyed peas = 33
Green beans = 31
Kidney beans = 29
Lentils = 29
Dried soybeans = 15

6. Sugars are found naturally in many foods. Sucrose and glucose (table sugar), fructose (fruits and vegetables), lactose (milk products), and maltose (flours and cereals) are all naturally occurring sugars. What you have to watch out for is *added* sugar; these are sugars that manufacturers add to foods during processing or packaging. Foods containing

fruit-juice concentrates, invert sugar, regular corn syrup, honey or molasses, hydrolyzed lactose syrup, or high-fructose corn syrup (made out of highly concentrated fructose through the hydrolysis of starch) all have added sugars. Many people don't realize, however, that pure, *unsweetened* fruit juice is still a potent source of sugar, even when it contains no added sugar. Extra lactose, dextrose, and maltose are also contained in many of your foods. In other words, the products may have naturally occurring sugars anyway, and then *more* sugar is thrown in to enhance consistency, taste, and so on. With the exception of lactose, which breaks down into glucose and galactose, all of these added sugars break down into fructose and glucose during digestion. To the body, no one sugar is more nutritional than the other; everything is broken down into either single sugars (called monosaccharides) or double sugars (called disaccharides), which are carried to cells through the bloodstream. The best way to know how much sugar is in a product is to look at the nutritional label for carbohydrates.

However, *how fast* that sugar is broken down and enters the bloodstream greatly depends on the amount of fiber in your food, how much protein you've eaten, and how much fat accompanies the sugar in your meal.

Ultimately, all the sugars from the foods you eat wind up as glucose. Your body doesn't know whether the sugar started out as maltose from whole-grain breads or lactose from milk products. Glucose then travels through your bloodstream to provide energy. If you have enough energy already, the glucose is stored as fat, for later. Sugars and starches (in equal "doses") affect blood sugar differently because of the time frame involved in glucose conversion. Sugars are converted faster than starches, so it's important to discuss sugar conversion with your nutritionist or doctor before you embark on a low-fat diet.

Sugar is added to food because it can change consistencies of foods and, in some instances, act as a preservative, as in jams and jellies. Sugars can increase the boiling point or reduce the freezing point in foods; sugars can add bulk and density, make baked goods do wonderful things, including helping yeast to ferment. Sugar can also add moisture to dry foods, making them "crisp," or balance acidic tastes found in foods like tomato sauce or salad dressing. Invert sugar is used to prevent sucrose from crystallizing in candy, while corn syrup is used for the same purpose.

Since the 1950s, a popular natural sugar in North America has been fructose, which has replaced sucrose in many food products in the form of high fructose syrup (HFS), made from corn. HFS was developed in response to high sucrose prices, and is very cheap to make. In other parts of the world, the equivalent of high-fructose syrup is made from whatever starches are local, such as rice, tapioca, wheat, or cassava. According to the International Food Information Council in Washington, D.C., the average North American consumes about thirty-seven grams of fructose daily. Bottom line: Watch your sugar intake.

Table 4.3

How Your Food Breaks Down

Complex Carbohydrates (digest more slowly)

- fruit
- vegetables* (corn, potatoes, etc.)
- grains (breads, pastas, and cereals)
- legumes (dried beans, peas, and lentils)

*Note: The following vegetables and/or herbs are very low in calories: artichokes, asparagus, mushrooms, bean sprouts, okra, onions, parsley, peppers, radish, celery, rapini, cucumber, shallots, eggplant, endive, tomato, kohlrabi, and zucchini.

Simple Carbohydrates* (digest quickly)

- fruits/fruit juices
- sugars (sucrose, fructose, etc.)

- honey
- corn syrup
- sorghum
- date sugar
- molasses
- lactose

*Note: lemon and lime juice, artificial sweeteners, and clear coffee or tea do not count.

Proteins* (digest slowly)

- lean meats
- fatty meats
- poultry
- fish
- eggs
- low-fat cheese
- high-fat cheese
- legumes
- grains

*Note: Bouillon, broth, or consommé, garlic, vinegar, herbs and spices, Worcester sauce, uncreamed horseradish, and soy sauce do not add significant calories.

Fats (digest slowly)

- high-fat dairy products (butter or cream)
- oils (canola/corn/olive/safflower/sunflower)
- lard
- avocados
- olives
- nuts
- fatty meats

Fiber (delays the conversion of other foods into glucose; helps form bulk so you can pass stools easily)

- whole-grain breads
- cereals (i.e., oatmeal)
- all fruits

Fiber (continued)
- legumes (beans and lentils)
- leafy greens
- cruciferous vegetables (cauliflower, broccoli, Brussels sprouts)

"How Your Food Breaks Down" copyright 1997, 1999, 2001, M. Sara Rosenthal.

---

7. Consume many differently colored fruits and vegetables. For color variety, select at least three differently colored fruit and vegetables daily.

8. Put fruit and sliced veggies in an easy-to-use, easy-to-reach place (sliced vegetables in the fridge; fruit out on the table).

9. Keep frozen and canned fruit and vegetables on hand to add to soups, salad, or rice dishes.

10. When purchasing, keep in mind the following:

   - Whole milk is made up of 48 per cent calories from fat.
   - 2 per cent milk gets 37 per cent of its calories from fat.
   - 1 per cent milk gets 26 per cent of its calories from fat.
   - Skim milk is completely fat-free.
   - Cheese gets 50 per cent of its calories from fat, unless it's skim-milk cheese.
   - Butter gets 95 per cent of its calories from fat.
   - Yogurt gets 15 per cent of its calories from fat unless it's fat-free.

THE SKINNY

A very low-fat diet such as the Pritikin or Ornish diets is intended for people who are serious about reducing their risk of heart disease; it is not a diet for the "masses." Nonetheless, the Center for Science in the Public Interest rated a number of diets for the masses in 2000. Very low-fat diets were actually found to be acceptable, but were found to restrict some healthy foods, such as seafood, low-fat poultry, and calcium. For people with high triglycerides above 200, it was suggested to cut out some carbohydrates and replace them with unsaturated fats (see Chapter 8). A less-restricting diet than the Pritikin and Ornish diets is the Choose to Lose program by Ron and Nancy Goor. In general, Pritikin and Ornish were examined in this chapter because they are the most revered in low-fat gospel; they are also the most extreme. *A diet is considered low fat when it restricts calories from fat to below 30 per cent daily.* The average person can stay healthy with 30 per cent of their calories from fat, which I'll discuss in Chapter 8.

Although people are generally confused about which foods raise and lower cholesterol, and which diets do the trick, it's been proven that people who cut their saturated fat to 7 to 10 per cent of calories, add cholesterol-lowering fiber (the soluble fiber) such as beans, peas, corn, and oatmeal, and include moderate exercise (such as a forty-five-minute walk per day) *will definitely lower their cholesterol and cut their risk of heart disease.*

CHAPTER 5

A Good Look at Low-Carb Diets

The short answer to "Are low-carb diets healthy?" is no. The short answer to "Can I lose weight on a low-carb diet" is yes.

For the purposes of this book, a diet is considered "low carb" when it restricts daily calories from carbohydrates to about 5 per cent. The most popular low-carb diet is the Atkins diet, named after Robert Atkins, who first promoted it. There are several types of Atkins-like diets on the market, but new generation "low-carb" diets, such as the Zone, or newer "protein diets" are far more balanced, allowing for a more equal distribution of carbohydrates and fats; these are not "low-carb" diets but instead encourage people to eat fewer carbohydrates to achieve a balance. Therefore, I discuss these diets separately on page 109 in this chapter, under the category "Lower-Carb Diets." The enormous interest, however, in truly low-carb diets, and the popularity of the Atkins diet, is what this chapter focuses on.

Low-carbohydrate diets are the opposite of low-fat diets; they restrict carbohydrates (on which a healthy diet should be based) to about 5 per cent of daily intake, and encourage the consumption of mostly high-fat foods – the more saturated fat, the better. These diets are also known as high-protein diets or, in clinical circles, *ketogenic diets* because they trigger a condition, which is potentially dangerous to some, called ketosis. It occurs when your insulin hormone is shut down, forcing your liver to produce ketone bodies. You'll certainly lose weight while in ketosis, but living in a state of ketosis is not what nature intended for a healthy human body living in North America – even though promoters of low-carb diets will tell you otherwise.

DEFINING A LOW-CARB DIET

The most popular of the low-carb diets is the Atkins diet, which initially restricts your carbohydrate intake to about twenty grams a day for the first phase of the program – called the Induction phase. The Induction phase is designed to put you into ketosis as soon as possible, a fact that Dr. Atkins makes crystal clear. Atkins explains, at length, what ketosis is and how it is a perfectly natural process that allows you to safely burn all your adipose tissue – that is, your unsightly fat. After reading Atkins's persuasive introduction, no one can wait to get started on his appealing, high-fat diet that promises to correct what's wrong with your body: too much insulin.

Once you're in ketosis, you enter the second phase of the diet, where you are reintroducing a few carbohydrates into your diet within the second week. You're supposed to add carbohydrates to the diet until you stop losing weight, which means you have reached your "critical carb load."

Although the "critical carb load" is supposed to help you reach a balance, few people reach that balance, however; many become so constipated in the first phase they go off the diet. Bad breath is also induced by ketosis, and many obese people at high risk of a heart attack will seek out the diet but should not be consuming such high levels of saturated fat. Many people have a genetic condition that causes high triglycerides, a condition that usually cannot be controlled through diet alone; for these people, the Atkins diet can be life-threatening (while a Pritikin Diet has been shown, since the 1950s, to be life-saving).

In all fairness, Atkins does encourage all of his readers to seek out a full medical exam before going on the diet; however, few of the people who buy diet books bother with this crucial step, and just want to see results. The diet is appealing to people who failed to lose weight on a low-fat diet. Potential Atkins dieters are told that it is carbohydrates that drive blood sugar levels up, spiking insulin levels, which are responsible for increasing appetite, raising tri-glycerides, and ultimately leading to obesity, insulin resistance, and type 2 diabetes. Anyone who overeats simple carbs, as opposed to complex carbs, as discussed in Chapter 4, is certainly at risk for this process. But eliminating all carbs is not the solution, since so many are nutrient-rich and vital for a healthy diet. People who were hungry on low-fat diets (because they lacked the information about food variety necessary to have a balance of interesting complex carbohydrates) are told that, at last, this is the "no hunger" diet. You can eat all the high fat you want and lose weight too. The Atkins diet does not require that you exercise, but encourages it.

HOW KETOSIS WORKS

We need to have adequate energy stores in our body to live. A healthy diet is varied, and supplies enough carbohydrates for con-version into available glucose for energy; in this process the hormone insulin is necessary in order to make the glucose available to the body. Insulin is a hormone made by your *beta cells*, the insulin-producing cells within the *islets of Langerhans* – small islands of cells afloat in your *pancreas*, a beak-shaped gland situated behind the stomach. Simply put, insulin regulates blood-sugar levels by "knocking" on your cells' doors and announcing, "Sugar's here. Come and get it!" Your cells then open the doors to let sugar in from your bloodstream. That sugar is absolutely vital to your health, and provides you with the energy you need to function.

When your glucose stores are low, due to the absence of sufficient carbohydrates in the diet, your body will tap into your glycogen stores, a concentrated source of glucose made and stored in your liver. We have about a six- to ten-hour supply of glycogen. When this supply runs out, fatty acids are degraded in the liver and released into the bloodstream as "ketone bodies" or ketones. Ketones are an alternative source of energy your body makes out of fatty acids when it is "desperate" for energy. When you begin to make ketones, you are in a state of ketosis. In this state, you literally live off your own fat; you will, therefore, lose weight. *But is this is a good way to lose weight?* Starvation will also induce weight loss, after all, as would throwing up your meal, the method practiced by bulimics.

Ketosis also suppresses the appetite, which Atkins extols as another virtue. Basically, ketosis is a "survival mechanism" the body adopts, which is what gets us through periods of famine or food deprivation. High concentrations of uric acid are produced while you are in ketosis, which in some people can lead to gout; in all people, ketosis puts a strain on the kidneys. The question for an Atkins candidate is "Can your kidneys survive the diet?" It is even a question Atkins poses himself to the reader, cautioning all pregnant women and people with kidney problems to stay away from this diet.

Most people can exist in a state of ketosis for a short while without any health consequences. Most of us have been in ketosis without knowing it dozens of times; it's what happens to us when we have missed meals or not eaten regularly or properly.

The argument has been made that, because ketosis is a "natural state" the body goes into, it is therefore harmless. Many hunter-based cultures, in fact, were living in ketosis to survive, so how can it be bad? Furthermore, Atkins points out that animals in hibernation are also in ketosis.

The problem with this reasoning is that it's not in context. The most obvious flaw is that comparing us to hibernating animals is absurd. Many biological (and sociological!) differences exist between a modern human in North America and an animal in hibernation.

Traditional hunter-culture ketogenic diets were far from the Atkins diet of heavy cream sauces and cheeseburgers (without the bun). The original Inuit diet, for example, was ketogenic; it was a diet high in fatty whale meat, with virtually no plant-based foods. But whale fat is very rich in omega-3 oils, which raises good cholesterol, or HDL, levels and actually protected the Inuit from heart disease. Once a moratorium was placed on whale hunting, however, and the Inuit began eating a Western-based diet, noted for high intakes of beef and other saturated fats, their heart disease rates soared. Other hunter-based cultures that lived on high-protein diets in the past were eating animal meat of a much different fat composition. Traditional game meat was composed of roughly 3 to 4 per cent fat, unlike today's beef, which is about 30 per cent fat.

WHAT'S SO BAD ABOUT KETOSIS?

Ketosis, in theory, is not dangerous for most people in good health, with no other health problems (there is no research on long-term effects). But most people trying out the Atkins diet are not in that category; many are obese and are showing signs of cardiovascular disease, including hypertension. Since ketosis puts a strain on the kidneys, it can definitely be life-threatening for people who have weakened kidneys due to high blood pressure, diabetes, or poor circulation, a sign of cardiovascular disease. People who suffer from bladder infections also have weakened kidneys. Already, this list rules out a lot of people from trying the Atkins diet; yet few people flocking to Atkins are aware they are poor candidates. Few people even realize that the treatment for kidney disease or kidney dysfunction is to put someone on a *low-protein diet* – the opposite of an Atkins-like diet.

Even data on the effects of short-term ketosis on healthy people on the Atkins diet is worrisome. Healthy people with no known health problems other than obesity have reported the following in the Induction phase, which is the ketogenic phase:

- headaches;
- fatigue;
- nausea (may be a sign of kidney problems);
- dehydration (due to fluid loss, which the kidneys normally regulate; a sign that the kidneys are overloaded);
- dizziness;
- constipation (due to lack of fiber); and/or
- bad breath (ketosis produces an acidic, fruity breath that is unpleasant).

UNDERSTANDING YOUR KIDNEYS

Many people who want to lose weight on the Atkins diet minimize the widely publicized risk of "kidney strain" associated with ketosis. That's because few people truly understand what the kidneys do in the body. Kidneys are not exactly a topic that gets a lot of media coverage, unlike heart disease or various cancers. *But it's crucial to understand kidney function in order to make an informed decision about whether the Atkins diet is right for you.*

Kidneys are the public servants of the body. If they go on strike, you lose your water service, garbage pickup, and a few other services you don't even appreciate.

Kidneys regulate your body's water levels. When you have too much water, your kidneys remove it by dumping it into a large storage tank: your bladder. The excess water stays there until you're ready to "pee it out." If you don't have enough water in your body (or if you're dehydrated), your kidneys will retain the water for you to keep you balanced.

Kidneys also act as your body's sewage-filtration plant. They filter out all the garbage and waste that your body doesn't need and dump it into the bladder; this waste is then excreted into your urine. The two waste products your kidneys regularly dump are urea (the waste product of protein) and creatinine (waste products produced by the muscles). In people with high blood-sugar levels, excess sugar will get sent to the kidneys, and the kidneys will dump it into the bladder too, causing sugar to appear in the urine.

Kidneys also balance calcium and phosphate in the body, which are needed to build bones. Kidneys operate two little side businesses on top of all of this. They make hormones. One hormone, called renin, helps to regulate blood pressure. Another hormone, called erythropoietin, helps bone marrow make red blood cells.

If you are interested in the Atkins diet, you are probably severely overweight and therefore may have cardiovascular disease and/or high blood pressure, and/or high blood sugar. *This means you likely already have early signs of kidney disease but don't know it yet.* High blood pressure typically damages blood vessels in the kidneys, which interferes with their job performance. As a result, they won't be as efficient at removing waste or excess water from your body. And if you are experiencing poor circulation, which can also cause water retention, the problem is further aggravated. Yet many people attempt the Atkins diet in this state, which is quite dangerous.

Poor circulation, a classic problem in obese people or those with evidence of heart disease, may cause the kidneys to secrete too much renin, which is normally designed to regulate blood pressure, but in ketosis, increases it. All the extra fluid and the high blood pressure places a heavy burden on your heart – and your kidneys. If this situation isn't brought under control, you'd likely suffer from a heart attack before kidney failure, but kidney failure is inevitable.

If you suffer from high blood sugar (one in four people older than age forty-five do – which means you may have diabetes but don't know it), it can affect small blood vessels in the kidneys' filters (called the nephrons), which is what leads to a diabetes complication known as diabetic nephropathy. In the early stages of nephropathy, good, usable protein is secreted in the urine. That's a sign that the kidneys were unable to distribute usable protein to the body's tissues. (Normally, they would excrete only the waste product of protein – urea – into the urine.)

People with bladder problems should also not undertake this diet. When the bladder isn't emptied fully for a variety of reasons (such as damage to the nerves controlling the bladder), there is a sort of sewage backup in your body. The first place that sewage hits is your kidneys. Old urine floating around your kidneys isn't a healthy thing, and it is something that is badly aggravated by ketosis.

Women who have a history of urinary-tract infections don't fare so well in ketosis either. Repeated urinary-tract infections may be a sign that your urine is too sugary, which predisposes you to bacteria such as E. coli. A high-protein diet may increase your exposure to this bacteria.

You may not always realize early stages of kidney disease, as there are often no symptoms at all. A blood test that looks for creatinine levels is a good indicator. Creatinine is a waste product removed from the blood by healthy kidneys. A creatinine blood test greater than 1.2 for women and 1.4 for men is a sign of kidney disease. Another test, which looks for blood urea nitrogen (BUN), is also important; when the BUN "rises," so to speak, it's also a sign of kidney disease. Other, more sensitive tests that detect the level of kidney function include tests for creatinine clearance, glomerular filtration rate (GFR), and urine albumin.

WHY A HIGH-PROTEIN DIET IS BAD FOR WEAKENED KIDNEYS

Protein is normally a good thing; it builds, repairs, and maintains your body tissues, and also helps you to fight infections or to heal wounds. But as protein breaks down in the body, it forms urea, which is a waste product. The kidney normally flushes out urea. When it can't, urea builds up in the blood. So, cutting down on protein – rather than increasing your intake of protein – is necessary when you show signs of kidney disease. Whether you're on the Atkins diet or not, any of the following symptoms can be early warning signs of kidney disease:

- a bad taste in the mouth (sign of toxins building up);
- blood or pus in the urine (a sign of a kidney infection);
- burning or difficulty urinating (a sign of a urinary-tract infection);
- foamy urine (a sign of kidney infection);
- foul-smelling or cloudy urine (a sign of a urinary-tract infection);
- frequent urination (a sign of high blood sugar and/or urinary-tract infection);
- leg swelling or leg cramps (a sign of fluid retention);
- your doctor detects protein in your urine (a sign of microvascular problems); and/or
- puffiness around the eyes, swelling of hands and feet (sign of edema, or fluid retention).

A SAMPLE MENU

There are various versions of a high-protein, low-carbohydrate diet such as the Atkins. Most encourage large quantities of protein in unrestricted amounts, including red meat, fish, shellfish, poultry, eggs, and cheese. The following foods are discouraged: pasta, bread, potatoes, fruit, many vegetables, and any foods with large amounts of refined sugar. Overall, roughly 60 per cent of calories are from fat; 35 per cent from protein; and only 5 per cent from carbohydrates. Of the roughly twenty amino acids in human proteins, twelve are made by the body; these are called the non-essential amino acids. The other eight we need have to come from our diet; these are called essential amino acids, which comprise isoleucine, leucine, lysine, methionine, phenylalanine, threonine, tryptophan, and valine. All protein foods containing all essential amino acids come from animal sources. Plant proteins are usually deficient in one or more of the essential amino acids, but that's normally taken care of by combining plants with one another, such as eating corn with beans. High-protein diets such as the Atkins exceed the recommended intake of protein by about four times; as we have seen, protein intake above the recommended requirement is not used properly by the body and places a burden on the kidneys and liver.

To get a better idea of what these diets look like in terms of a daily meal plan, here's a sneak preview.

A typical breakfast would be bacon and eggs with no toast or juice. Lunch might be a double cheeseburger with no bun and a small salad with a high-fat dressing. Dinner might be steak or fried chicken with another salad topped with a high-fat dressing. No alcohol or caffeine are allowed, and no desserts are allowed either.

This is a "be careful what you wish for" diet. People often wind up eating no more than about 1,200 to 1,500 calories per day – the same as in a low-fat diet – because they can eat only so much fat before they feel sick.

PROS AND MORE CONS

The benefits of this diet are that, if your kidneys can survive ketosis (likely so long as you do not have the conditions outlined earlier – conditions that frequently accompany obesity), you will indeed lose weight, not feel hungry, and will eat very little sugar or white flour. Essentially, you will self-regulate to a diet that is actually quite low in calories. The weight loss you experience could correct other problems, such as high cholesterol and insulin resistance. Indeed, it's been long known by diabetes experts that even a small weight loss can help to reverse insulin resistance.

That said, if high blood sugar or high cholesterol was a problem you had going into the Atkins diet, you risked ruining your kidneys in ketosis for the same weight-loss benefits you could have found on any low-calorie diet, including a balanced one, such as those in Chapter 8.

Nutrition experts maintain that weight loss on the Atkins diet is achieved due to better compliance: you like the diet better, so you stick to it. In other words, reducing calories will always equal weight loss; you don't have to go into ketosis to do that!

The downsides of this diet are numerous. Aside from the risk to the kidneys outlined earlier, a diet high in saturated fat can raise

LDL cholesterol levels, normally counterbalanced by foods high in fiber such as fruits and vegetables. Also, high blood pressure can ensue when people are denied a variety of fruits and vegetables, which are normally rich sources of potassium, calcium, and magnesium – known to regulate blood pressure. High "sat fat" diets are also high in sodium, known to raise blood pressure. In addition, high-protein foods such as meat, poultry, and seafood are high in purines, substances that are broken down into uric acid and can cause gout in some people. Too much protein in the body increases calcium lost through the urine, predisposing you to osteoporosis. Without sufficient carbohydrates, fatigue often sets in too.

People on this diet are often reluctant to – or won't – feed their children the same food they're eating, which is a major sign that this is not a diet that is sustainable for good health. Aside from getting tired, most find that the allure of high fats wears rather thin; the diet gets "tired" after a while, and many people complain of feeling ill after only a couple of weeks. (We are genetically designed to crave variety.) The diet is, contrary to what most people believe, very difficult to stick to in restaurants – even more difficult than a low-fat diet at times. You constantly have to remove the carbohydrates from your dishes, which, after all, are provided in most restaurants for balance.

WHAT THE CRITICS SAY

The instinct to eat a variety of foods is within us. We needed to survive by eating a range of nutrients: protein, fat, and carbohydrates, which are primarily made up of essential nutrients such as grains, fruits, and vegetables. The central criticism of this diet is that it dramatically reduces, if not eliminates, the macronutrient most essential to the human body: carbohydrates.

The Center for Science in the Public Interest rates low-carbohydrate diets such as Atkins, Protein Power, and Sugar Busters as unacceptable because of the high quantities of saturated

fat and low quantities of fiber and essential nutrients that they recommend. People become constipated, and may burn fat due to
ketosis, but at the same time they are depriving their bodies of
essential nutrients, many of which are known to decrease incidences of diseases such as certain cancers. People who are loading
their bodies with saturated fats known to be associated with
higher rates of cancers are obviously putting themselves at risk.
Worse, in some individuals with genetically caused high cholesterol
and high triglycerides, consuming high levels of saturated fats can
be life-threatening. Critics are careful to point out that people are
not just eating "saturated fat" when they are encouraged to load up
on fast foods either. As discussed in Chapter 1, most fast food is so
overprocessed and full of trans fatty acids and chemical residue, it
is difficult to know exactly what one is eating when one is told to
"go forth unto a burger joint and eat all you want." There are
many hidden ingredients in high-fat foods.

Sound nutritional experts maintain that carbohydrates do not
make us fat; it is overindulgence in carbohydrates – especially simple
carbohydrates – or protein or fat that makes us fat. Eating less carbs,
protein, and fat – in other words, eating everything in moderation,
and expending more energy than is consumed, is the key to weight
loss. Eating whole-grain breads and cereals, pasta, rice, potatoes,
beans, and fruit and vegetables do not make us fat; eating candy,
chocolate, cookies, biscuits, sweets, and cakes – all of which are
refined carbohydrates – make us fat. And that is discouraged on any
balanced diet. In short, any balanced diet will result in weight loss
with the added benefit of being healthy.

Low-carb/high-protein diets also run counter to the dietary
guidelines set forth by the World Cancer Research Fund, which I
discussed in Chapter 3.

Reams of anecdotal research reveal that many people cannot
survive the Induction phase of the Atkins diet. They see no
improvement in their cholesterol levels either, and some find they
worsen. Those that do see improvement are likely seeing improvement due to weight loss resulting from simply eating fewer calories.

Most scholarly and experienced nutrition experts maintain that basic dietary advice hasn't changed over the last fifty years: a calorie is a calorie. Eat fewer calories and you'll lose weight. This is why a low-fat diet, when followed correctly, works too.

The American Heart Association's Nutrition Committee of the Council on Nutrition, Physical Activity and Metabolism asserts that there are no long-term studies to back up any of Atkins' claims. Again, it asserts that beneficial effects on cholesterol levels or insulin levels are due to weight loss, not the process by which the weight was lost. The illusion of greater weight loss, according to the AHA, is due to fluid loss related to reduced carbohydrate intake and ketosis-induced appetite suppression. Although the initial weight loss may be quite fast, it is probably not sustained, because it lacks the main ingredient of long-term sustainability: balance.

A flurry of recent short-term studies on the Atkins diet (published in 2002 and 2003) have found that the diet works well for some people because it winds up, at the end of the day, being a low-calorie diet. Obesity researchers doing small-sample studies on Atkins dieters are finding that, on average, they are losing about twice as much weight than people on balanced diets that are called "low fat" but are not at all the same diets Ornish and Pritikin promote for reversing heart disease. In these studies, the calories from fat were roughly 20 per cent, twice the amount of fat found with Ornish, for example. The appearance of greater weight loss with the Atkins diet is, again, due to fluids lost during ketosis. But Atkins dieters in some studies demonstrate a rise in their bad cholesterol levels (LDL) as well as their good cholesterol levels. This is likely due to the fact that good fats were ingested on Atkins along with bad fats. But this is now the norm amongst balanced diets that don't risk your health, such as the Mediterranean diet in Chapter 6.

On the low-fat diets in which 20 per cent of calories were from fat, bad cholesterol did drop, but good cholesterol remained about the same. This means that no bad fats were added to the diet, and cholesterol was slowly improving. Other studies of the Atkins diet have found, however, that the cholesterol levels remained the same. This is what is meant by headlines on the news regarding "new studies show Atkins diet works." However, once you really look at the biology behind these studies, the results are far from "stunning."

There is in fact a body of literature on ketogenic diets that supports the notion that the Atkins diet works because of calorie reduction, pure and simple. The only people who are medically advised to go on ketogenic diets are certain children who have seizures; for reasons not well understood, diets that are about 80 per cent fat seem to suppress seizures in children who do not respond well to anti-seizure medications. Long-term studies on these children suggest that they lost and gained weight according to the number of calories they ate, in spite of the fact that they were in a constant state of ketosis.

The most telling study that would vindicate Atkins is the one that cannot be done: no study has compared Atkins to Ornish or Pritikin, which would actually compare apples to apples. The reason is because anyone with the risk factors high enough to warrant a Pritikin or Ornish diet would not survive ketosis because of the kidney damage that would likely follow. No one has studied the effect of long-term ketosis on Atkins dieters, either, which would shed much more light on the overall safety of Atkins for people wanting to lose weight who were in otherwise good health. Calorie for calorie, the Atkins diet is actually nothing but a low-calorie diet in a souped-up package.

OTHER LOWER-CARB DIETS

Standard guidelines recommend that people should be getting about 50 to 55 per cent of their calories from carbohydrates, which many nutritionists argue are too much. If you're interested in a *lower*-carb diet, that is a kinder, gentler Atkins, you can try the Zone or the South Beach Diet. The Zone is deemed acceptable by nutritionists – but not for the "pseudoscientific" reasons offered by Barry Spears, creator of the Zone. The Zone refers to the "hormonal zone" in which insulin levels are minimized due to lower intake of carbohydrates. Is it true? Probably some truth and some spin is within the Zone theory. Few really understand it, however, as the Zone is terribly technical and close to impossible for the average person to truly comprehend. But who cares? Nutritionists explain that the Zone is a safe diet because it is simply *a balanced diet*. The 40:30:30 balance the Zone encourages, for example, is simply a reasonable low-calorie balanced diet, and that is what's behind the weight loss. Although it's a bit too low in grains and calcium, at least you have enough fruit and vegetables and are not being deprived of nutrients. The ratio 40:30:30 refers to the balance of macronutrients in each meal; the Zone encourages that you get 40 per cent of your calories from carbs; 30 per cent from protein, and 30 per cent from fat. There's nothing wrong with that. When you buy into the Zone, you're buying a balanced, low-calorie diet in a shiny new package. But people who are on the Zone are not on a diet that is considered "low carb" by more extreme standards.

As for the South Beach Diet, created by Dr. Arthur Agatson, it is essentially a balanced diet that eliminates "bad carbs" and "bad fats" such as cakes, cookies, and "white stuff" (white bread, white rice, potatoes). In the first fourteen days of the diet, you are also forbidden to have alcohol, and any sugar – including fruits. After fourteen days, most things can be reintroduced in moderation. The "buzz" over this diet is the dramatic weight loss of roughly eight to thirteen pounds in the first two weeks, due, of course, to the elimination of very fattening foods. Losing weight in the abdominal area (the adipose tissue) is particularly successful on this diet, which the diet's creator attributes to the elimination of insulin-producing foods such as simple carbs. Critics have noted that the weight loss is more likely due to loss of "water weight," which occurs in any diet that eliminates hundreds of calories a day from the "bad foods." The South Beach Diet is touted for being neither a low-carb nor low-fat diet, but the "right diet." Indeed, it emphasizes all of the "good fats" and "good carbs" discussed in Chapter 7 and 8. Again, it's a balanced diet in a shiny new package!

THE SKINNY

The Atkins diet is not considered worth the risk for what you get: a 1,500-calorie diet that deprives you of essential nutrients, potentially kills you with saturated fat, and may put you at risk for certain cancers known to be associated with high levels of saturated fat. Recent studies also show an association between diets high in saturated fat and Alzheimer's disease. You can get a healthful 1,500-calorie diet from a number of programs that don't put your health at risk. If you're overweight and otherwise healthy (your blood sugar, blood pressure, and blood fats are all normal rather than even slightly elevated), you'll probably survive it, but it's not a diet that anyone can promote as one you can use for life, and it's certainly not a diet you can promote for children or teens, which is telling indeed. Meanwhile, even an extreme Ornish or Pritikin diet is fine for everyone, when followed correctly, and there are absolutely no health consequences other than improved health.

CHAPTER 6

THE OLIVE AND THE VINE:

The Mediterranean Diet and the French Paradox

Whenever health problems linked to diet and obesity began to be scrutinized in the 1960s and 1970s, much of the research was clinical, analyzing dietary components that were unhealthy. But one of the most interesting research approaches was "epidemiological" – which involves looking at more cultural and geographical parts of the dietary puzzle. Over time, researchers observed that people who lived in Mediterranean countries, such as Greece and Italy, were healthier than North Americans, in spite of the fact that they ate a lot of pasta and olive oil. And thus began intense interest in what we in the West refer to as the Mediterranean diet, sometimes known as the olive-oil diet, which is not so much a diet that someone invented but a way of eating that has become known as a diet of sorts.

Other epidemiological research revealed that people living in France had less heart disease, in spite of a diet heavy in saturated fat. The noted difference in the French diet was the incorporation of red wine daily into the meal. Studies that looked into health benefits of red wine also became an interest for many, and this chapter also focuses on that.

The terms *good fats* and *bad fats* began to crystallize around the late 1980s, when the research done into diets higher in mono-unsaturated fats were looked at closely. It was found that, in spite of the fact that they were "fats," they raised good cholesterol (HDL), which protects against heart disease. The Mediterranean diet, in particular, has been dependent upon olive oil for almost all its dishes. Olive oil is used on salads, hot vegetables, in pasta sauces, or poured plain onto pastas with a little garlic. Olive oil, herbs, and spices are routinely used in place of butter as spreads or dips for breads. According to the study, properties of olive oil were found to contain a host of protective factors and "catalyst" ingredients that allowed phytochemicals from plant-based foods to work their magic in the body. The virtues of a Mediterranean diet with its "good fats" became the basis for a revolution in dietary-fat guidelines, which now recognize that healthy diets should have some monounsaturated fats, the best of which is olive oil.

Around this same time French researchers wondered why, with the French diet being so high in saturated fat, the rates of heart disease among the French were so much lower than in Britain and North Americans, where the diets were also high in saturated fats? This was dubbed the French Paradox, and investigators began to look more closely at the French diet, a diet that seemed to be filled with "bad fats" – creams, butter, fois gras – all saturated fats, saturated in even *more* saturated fats. But then there was a key difference: the French drank red wine with their meals. Studies began to look at whether moderate drinking – such as red wine sipped with meals – contributed to lower rates of heart disease. They found that it did, but only in moderation. (The Mediterranean diet, of course, is also based on regular-yet-moderate consumption of red wine.) Suddenly, the Olive and the Vine became the focus of a flurry of "fat" and heart-disease research.

This chapter explores the cuisine or menu, and epidemiology, of French and Mediterranean diets. The French Paradox, as it turns out, is not so much a paradox but an error in statistical analysis, with a few key cultural differences in eating behavior overlooked. Nonetheless, the health benefits of moderate red-wine drinking, combined with olive-oil-based diets, are real. You can create a wonderful, balanced diet with these ingredients. And that's a diet you can keep for life, as will be discussed in Chapter 8.

THE OLIVE

Forget the creamed spinach! Even Popeye knew that the best thing for his spinach-eating was his true love, Olive Oyl. The Mediterranean diet has been dubbed "the healthiest diet in the world." Many controlled studies that placed one group of people on a Mediterranean diet for two years or more, and a regular North American diet for that time frame, found that the heart-disease rates dropped dramatically in the Mediterranean group. Olive oil, rich in linolenic and oleic acids, vitamins E, and antioxidants; garlic; fresh fruits and vegetables; and relatively lower meat consumption are considered to be most of the story. Although wine drinking is an important component of the Mediterranean diet, as it was of the French, the Mediterranean diet is no paradox. Saturated-fat consumption is low, and mono-unsaturated consumption is high, which elevates and thus protects against heart disease. The wine does not account for the differences in heart-disease rates; the type of fats consumed does.

WHAT IS A MEDITERRANEAN DIET?

The Mediterranean diet refers to diets within olive-growing regions of the Mediterranean, which explains the heavy reliance on olive oil. But if you look at the components of a healthy diet (see Chapter 8), the Mediterranean approach has them all: a large consumption of salads and legumes, whole grains (wheat), olives (whole), grapes, other fruits, including wine. The total fat consumption in a Mediterranean diet is higher than our fat guidelines in North America: around 40 per cent in some regions, such as Greece and Spain, where fish is eaten more, but right on target – about 30 per cent – in Italy.

In Chapter 8, I refer to physician Ancel Keys, who pioneered international heart-study research as early as 1947, when he noticed a sharp rise in heart disease in the United States. When he travelled to Italy in 1952, he observed the Mediterranean diet and concluded that it was the healthiest diet in the world, calling it the "good Mediterranean diet." His heart-healthy dietary guidelines, based on the findings of his Italy trip, were published in 1959 in his book *How to Eat and Stay Well the Mediterranean Way*. In the late 1950s, Keys and his colleagues undertook a fifteen-year project in which they collected data on more than 12,000 men from seven countries – Finland, Greece, Italy, Japan, Yugoslavia, the Netherlands, and the United States. It was known as the Seven Country Study, and its results were published in 1984. Keys noted that the lowest rates of heart disease in the world were in Mediterranean countries, notably Greece, and the second-lowest were in Japan; yet Japan's heart-disease rate was still twice that of Greece's. In 1986, a followup analysis on the Seven Country Study found that intakes of monounsaturated fat, such as olive oil, were the reason for such low heart-disease rates.

Keys took note of Greece's high olive-oil consumption and low saturated-fat consumption. He recorded olive-oil consumption as high as 20 kg/person/year, compared to France's consumption, which was far lower. In Greece, the olive tree is associated with peace, because it takes olive trees thirty years to mature and bear olives; thus, legend has it, the trees were only planted in Greece when society was stable.

The major fatty acid in olives is oleic acid, a monounsaturated fatty acid comprising 56 to 83 per cent of olive oil. The polyunsaturated fatty acids in olive oil are represented by the omega-6 fatty acid, linoleic (3.5 to 20 per cent), and the omega-3 fatty acid, alpha-linolenic (0 to 1.5 per cent). Fatty fish are also high in omega-3 fatty acids, but olive oil provides all the good fats you need without going fishing! Studies confirm that, when you replace saturated fats with monounsaturated (such as olive oil) or polyunsaturated fat, you can preserve HDL cholesterol levels better and lower both your total cholesterol and bad cholesterol (LDL).

Other monounsaturated oils are canola, peanut, sesame, soybean, corn, cottonseed, and safflower, but olive oil is 74 per cent monounsaturated, while the next-best oil, canola, is only 59 per cent monounsaturated. Olive oil also makes the carotenes in vegetables come alive, while non-fat dressings or no-monounsaturated oils on salad actually make the salad's nutrients inferior by blocking their absorption. Carotenes are lipophilic, meaning "fat loving." If you don't consume fat along with carotenes within a couple of hours, you won't absorb any of the nutrients they have to offer. While any fat will do on carotenes, olive oil, being heart protective, is the best option. In fact, dressing your salads with olive oil is one of the best ways to protect your heart.

Oily fish that are high in polyunsaturated omega-3 fatty acids are also part of the Mediterranean diet, as are nuts, garlic, and snails. In short, if we're well oiled, we'll apparently run better and resist "rust." Olive oil literally helps to offset oxidation, which is a natural process in the body that leads to cell breakdown. That's why antioxidants are considered so valuable in cancer prevention.

The only hole you can poke in the Mediterranean diet studies – which all point to the same conclusion: yep, olive oil is great for our health – is that other factors such as lifestyle (more activity, less depression due to a more community-oriented society, or plain genetics) could be operating in the countries of the Mediterranean. But studies on North Americans who have adopted the Mediterranean diet confirm the same health benefits.

IS THIS A "DIET"?

In North America, we don't think of our eating habits as "regional"; we tend to look for the "best diet" all the time. In cultures with traditional diets with the same staple ingredients for centuries, the diet is simply a way of life – which is what the word *diet* means, from the Greek root, *diaita*. People in Greece or Italy or Spain just eat; they don't talk about "diets" and dieting. Although we may notice the components of the Mediterranean diet as "carbs, protein, and fats" – people there don't tend to buy dietary components: *they buy food.*

Those interested in trying out the Mediterranean diet will find that it's not that different from what you already eat and are exposed to. A typical daily menu plan from such a diet looks something like this. Breakfast would be pretty close to what you might already have: a high-fiber granola, or a hot cereal with fruit and skim milk. Or a couple of soft-boiled eggs on whole-wheat toast (they can be poached or hard-boiled, or fried in a non-stick pan). You can have plain yogurt with fruit, or toast with jam. Lunch could be a big salad, with olive oil and vinegar dressing (1/4 cup vinegar to 3/4 olive oil with herbs and spices as you wish). Lunch also might consist of a lentil soup with bread dipped in olive oil or one of the following with a fruit: roast-pepper-and-cheese sandwich, pasta salads (cooked pasta with vegetables and the olive-oil dressing), potato salad (same as pasta salad only with potatoes); tuna salad (substitute the mayo for the olive-oil dressing); a baked potato (substitute olive oil and salt for the butter and sour cream). Dinner might consist of any grilled or broiled fish, shrimp, seafood, or chicken, seasoned with olive oil and spices; a baked potato with olive oil and salt instead of butter and sour cream; and a salad with olive-oil dressing and some feta cheese. Or you can grill or broil any vegetable (fresh or frozen), lightly brushed with olive oil, which makes them delicious. Instead of meat or fish, you can make any type of pasta with a marinara (tomato-based) sauce, or a sauce of olive oil, garlic, and herbs. You could add some meat or vegetables to the pasta as well. You could have bread dipped in olive oil to go with it. Fruit for dessert, a glass of red wine with dinner. There are hundreds of things you can make easily. When shopping for a Mediterranean meal plan, it is best to stock up on: frozen vegetables, beans and legumes (for soups especially), some cheeses such as feta, parmesan, romano, or provolone (you can buy these all as non-fat cheeses); seafood, such as canned clams for marinara sauces; fruits; garlic; red wine or grape juice; poultry, game, and fish of your choice; lemons; salad fixings; mushrooms, olives, and olive oil (of course); balsamic vinegar; rice; peppers (for roasting); spinach; tomatoes; tuna; and yogurt. Get yourself a Mediterranean cookbook with plenty of Italian and Greek recipes, and you should be able to eat interesting foods without getting tired or bored. Most women do well on about 1,500 calories per day, and men on about 2,000 calories per day.

WALKING MEDITERRANEAN STYLE

In Italy, the *passeggiata* is the "daily stroll" around a neighborhood or shopping area. It lasts for about an hour and is usually with a friend or family member, window shopping, buying certain foods for dinner, and so forth. We North Americans can do this easily in most cities. If you live in a suburban area of strip malls, plan a walk around the neighborhood, walk your dog, etc. Regardless of what you decide to do for your daily activity, substitute a walk for something else: a bike ride, dancing lessons, etc. The point is that the Mediterranean diet incorporates about an hour of moderate activity per day – which used to be just part of everyone's life.

PROPERTIES OF OLIVE OIL

Olive oil contains a wealth of phytochemicals (plant chemicals) and micronutrients. They include the following, all of which prevent oxidation:

- caffeic acid;
- ferulic acid;
- hydroxytyrosol;
- oleuropien;
- squaline;
- vitamin E; and
- vanillic acid (a polyphenol, which is also found in wine).

THE VINE

When news of the French Paradox and red-wine drinking was broadcast on *60 Minutes* in November 1991, sales of red wine skyrocketed as did the prices of wine. But studies were not able to show, conclusively, that moderate wine drinking was any better than moderate intake of any alcohol, although naturally, the wine industry began funding more research into studies that looked at specific properties of red wine, and how these might affect blood cholesterol and overall rates of heart disease. Much of this research supported that moderate drinking – defined as two drinks per day for men, and one drink per day for women – was not harmful and was potentially healthful in that it was associated with lowering cholesterol levels. The American 1990 guidelines regarding alcohol consumption had stated: "Drinking has no benefits" and did not recommend any alcohol. By 1995, U.S. alcoholic guidelines read: "Alcoholic beverages have been used to enhance the enjoyment of meals by many societies throughout human history." No health claim was made, but, nonetheless, it was implied. The wine industry was now anxious to begin promoting wine as a health food for its own gain. But because moderate drinking can so easily cross into alcohol abuse, health claims about red wine are difficult to make. By 2000, the U.S. guidelines made it clear that excess alcohol consumption was harmful; this made it impossible for the wine industry to quote guidelines on their labels. But few people truly understand what the studies really show about red wine and cholesterol.

THE WINE STUDIES

As early as 1979, French researchers demonstrated a relationship between low rates of heart disease and wine, in spite of diets rich in saturated fats. The most comprehensive study that appears to have solved the French Paradox was not a wine study per se but an international study looking at heart-disease rates around the world, including rates of heart disease in France and Mediterranean countries. Known as the WHO MONICA Project (World Health Organization Monitoring of Trends and Determinants in Cardiovascular Disease), this was a ten-year study that monitored deaths from heart disease and risk factors in men and women from ages thirty-five to sixty-four in various communities between 1985 and 1987, and was inspired by Keys's Seven Country Study. This project found major differences in the incidence of heart disease and death rates, a surprising finding given that there were even differences in regions with common diets, such as those of France, Britain, and the United States. MONICA was the study that began the French Paradox; it also confirmed data from the Seven Country Study regarding low rates of heart disease in Mediterranean countries. MONICA led some investigators to look at the properties in olive oil and garlic, while others looked at properties in wine.

Throughout the 1990s, more convincing evidence regarding red wine began to appear. The Copenhagen City Heart Study was another good examination of wine and heart disease. Published in 1998, it followed wine drinkers for ten to twelve years and found that moderate wine drinking, rather than the consumption of beer or spirits, was associated with a lower risk of stroke.

RED PROPERTIES

Some researchers joked that dissecting red-wine properties seemed useless, since whatever magic it conferred was in the best form already. Nonetheless, red-wine property studies ensued, and many things were uncovered as a result. For example, anthocyanin, which gives red wine and black olives their color, was postulated to have antioxidant effects, as were a host of "disease-fighting compounds" known as polyphenols, such as quercetin, also found in tea, onions, and apple skin. One of the most noted compounds of red wine is resveratrol, whose only other source is peanuts. Since it is known to have a greater antioxidant activity than vitamin E, researchers at the University of Omaha claim that resveratrol is a "super antioxidant" in red grapes.

Red wine is believed to have a heart-healthy effect in three ways: it is antioxidant, vasodilating, and antithrombotic (that is, it decreases the likelihood of clots forming in blood). The two most studied compounds in wine are resveratrol and quercitin. Resveratrol also apparently increases HDL cholesterol by preventing LDL cholesterol from oxidating. The tannins in red wine, which are not as present in white wine or other liquor, seem to help blood flow and declog arteries. In fact, studies find that even half a bottle of red wine per night does no harm – other than adding about 250 calories to your meal.

But many of the wine studies are narrow in focus: they look at properties in wine that do various things in test tubes or to rats and mice, and indirectly apply it to human beings with statements such as (and I sweepingly paraphrase dozens of studies here): "More research is needed, but resveratrol positively affects cholesterol in mice." A lot of these types of laboratory studies get misinterpreted on the evening news as: "And today, another study published about red wine shows it can prevent heart disease." These types of studies are not as meaningful as studies that actually compared rates of heart disease and stroke in non-wine drinkers to wine drinkers. One significant large study found that there were no differences in heart disease between people who drank only red wine or only white wine.

De-alcoholized red wine as well as purple grape juice may also have the same benefits as red wine. One study used purple grape juice instead of red wine in people with heart disease, and found their cholesterol levels improved.

WHAT'S IN THAT WINE?

The following properties of red wine, which may or may not contribute to heart health, have been found in laboratory studies:

- Anthocyanin. A flavonoid that provides the red pigment in grapes, and has been found to be an antioxidant that also may inhibit cholesterol production and prevent blood clots.
- Caffeic acid. An antioxidant, also found in olive oil.
- Catechin. A flavonoid that may reduce bad cholesterol and decrease blood clotting.
- Cinnamic acid. A polyphenol that may inhibit the growth of cancer cells.
- Ellagic acid. Helps prevent oxidation.
- Epicatechin. Helps inhibit oxidation.
- Ferulic acid. Inhibits oxidation, also found in olive oil.
- Gentisic acid. An Aspirin-like compound found in red wine. An antioxidant, anti-inflammatory, and antibacterial.
- Leucocyanidol. May help reduce inflammation of the blood vessels associated with heart disease.
- P-coumaric. Another polyphenol.
- Polydatin. Helps inhibit platelet formation and clotting.
- Quercetin. An antioxidant that helps reduce clotting.
- Resveratrol. A flavonoid that inhibits oxidation and reduces platelet stickiness. Has also been shown to inhibit tumor growth in certain cancers.

- Salicylic acid. Closely related to acetylsalicylic acid, or Aspirin, which people take to reduce blood clots.
- Tannic acid. Helps to dilate blood vessels.
- Taxifolin. Helps inhibit lipid oxidation.
- Vanillic acid. Antibacterial and antifungal.

NO FRENCH PARADOX?

As the wine research continued throughout the 1980s, researchers looking more carefully at the MONICA study raised a more shocking possibility: Perhaps there was no French Paradox. The "time lag" theory was introduced as an explanation for the French Paradox. Researchers analyzing the results of MONICA found that a serious error had been made, which may have accounted for the French Paradox. The French diet has only recently become as filled with saturated fat. Not enough time had elapsed in France for the changes in their diet to catch up with mortality rates. Researchers compared the French Paradox from MONICA to introducing cigarettes for the first time to a large country and not waiting long enough for the lung cancer to show up.

Britain and the United States, which had been compared with France, had been consuming red meat in large quantities for decades. Meat consumption in large quantities in France occurred only recently. Saturated fats from meats are also different than saturated fats from cheeses or other dairy products. France was largely a rural society until the 1950s, when it began to recover from the Second World War; people ate less because they were poor. It was not until the 1970s that France's saturated-fat consumption started to truly compare to Britain and the United States. Prior to 1970, the French were consuming a diet that supplied roughly 21 per cent of their calories from fat – which is a relatively low-fat diet. Moreover, in North America, children begin consuming a diet high in saturated fat before children in France do. This also has bearing on future heart-disease rates. In order to do a truly comparative study, we would have to wait to see what the effects of the 1980s diet has on France's fifty-plus generation. The heart-disease rates in France found by the MONICA study were probably based on the pre-1970s diet. In fact, MONICA revealed the same French heart-disease rates as the Seven Country Study, which was done throughout the 1960s and early 1970s, and was thus also based on that diet that got 21 per cent of calories from fat.

Other explanations for the French Paradox were that not all deaths from heart disease were accurately recorded as being caused by heart disease. Instead, complications of heart disease were often cited as the cause of death, which affects the data.

It's also noted that, in countries where wine drinking is prevalent, other drinks are not. Wine is cheaper in many European countries than water or soft drinks or juice; in addition, France, Italy, and Spain all shared low consumption of saturated fat until recently.

Even if a MONICA study were repeated, heart-disease deaths have also gone down due to better medications for lowering cholesterol and hypertension. For example, in 1993, 34 per cent of survivors of heart attacks in France took cholesterol-lowering drugs compared with 4 per cent of survivors in Britain; 63 per cent of French took Aspirin compared with 38 per cent in Britain; another 20 per cent took anticoagulants, compared with 5 per cent in Britain.

Another key difference in obesity and heart-disease rates is that fast food has not infiltrated France as much as it has Britain and the United States. This makes a huge difference in cultural eating patterns.

THE FRENCH ATTITUDE TO FOOD: ANOTHER EXPLANATION FOR THE PARADOX

The French have a saying, which is derived from the lyrics of an old French torch song: "Regret nothing – in matters of love and food." Researchers also looked at French attitudes to food and found that it may explain some of the paradox too. One study that compared food attitudes between North American eaters and French eaters uncovered a vast difference in eating patterns and beliefs about food. In short, the French are passionate about their food and really enjoy it. They never think of food as "sinful"; instead, they simply think of it as "tasty." To the French, food is a work of art, meant to be enjoyed. To the North American, food is "calories" and "fattening" and "forbidden." North Americans tend to think about food as either fuel or poison; they fear the effect food will have on their bodies. In France, good food feeds the *soul*, not the body. (Apparently, General de Gaulle used to say, "It's difficult to govern a country that has five hundred varieties of cheese.") In France, the idea of "food police" watching every gram of fat is mocked. What is also mocked is the way in which North Americans eat: everywhere and anywhere is a dining room. We eat in our cars, while walking on the street, and at our desks when we work. In France, eating takes place at restaurants or at dinner tables. The North American pattern of eating is considered by the French to be nomadic eating, or vagabond feeding and grazing. There is also a huge distinction between quantity and quality of food. In North America, we are taught that large portions are good – even if the food is mediocre and of poor quality. In France, the quality and taste of the food is the most important factor, and when taste is there, and the quality of the food is high, the appetite is satiated, and the quantity or portion size is not important. The French may, in fact, be simply eating less than North Americans, even though they are eating diets high in saturated fats. This supports, again, the notion that eating less – no matter what it is – may be where the real health benefits come in. It also supports the "time lag" theory discussed earlier.

CALORIES AND ALCOHOL

Imbibe, by all means! But alcohol, it should be remembered, is fattening, delivering about 7 calories per gram, or 150 calories per drink. A glass of dry red or white wine has calories but no sugar. The same thing goes for cognac, brandy, and dry sherry that contain no sugar.

On the other hand, a sweet wine listed as (3) in Ontario or British Columbia means that it contains 3 grams of sugar per 100 mL, or one 3.5-ounce portion. Dessert wines or ice wines are really sweet; they contain about 15 per cent sugar, or 10 grams of sugar for a 2-ounce serving. Sweet liqueurs are 35 per cent sugar.

A glass of dry wine with your meal adds about 100 calories. Half soda water and half wine (a spritzer) contains half the calories. When you cook with wine, the alcohol evaporates, leaving only the flavor.

If you're a beer drinker, that's about 150 calories per bottle; a light beer has fewer calories but contains at least 100 calories per bottle.

The stiffer the drink, the fatter it gets. Hard liquors such as scotch, rye, gin, and rum are made out of cereal grains; vodka, the Russian staple, is made out of potatoes. In this case, the grains ferment into alcohol. Hard liquor averages about 40 per cent alcohol, but has no sugar. Nevertheless, you're looking at about 100 calories per small shot glass, so long as you don't add fruit, tomato, or clamato juice, or sugary soft drinks.

THE SKINNY

It's well established that a Mediterranean diet is a good model for a diet for life, which can be incorporated into the ideas to be discussed in Chapter 8. Diets that use olive oil or a monounsaturated fat (remember, olive oil is 74 per cent monounsaturated) as the main source of dietary fat, along with whole grains, fruits, vegetables, and omega-3 fatty acids (also in olive oil), were stated to be, in a 2002 article in the *Journal of the American Medical Association*, "the optimal diet for prevention of heart disease." The article added that avoiding smoking and getting regular activity along with this diet may prevent the majority of heart disease in Western populations. That is a pretty strong endorsement for an olive-oil-based diet. Red wine, while not thought to be the reason behind the French paradox anymore, is nevertheless considered to be a healthy and natural way possibly to reduce cholesterol when consumed in moderation. If you can't drink wine for some reason, you can have grape juice or de-alcoholized wine, which apparently confer some of the same benefits as the alcoholic version.

CHAPTER 7

FAT PHARM

W hen discussing fat and diet, a crucial element is knowledge of the pharmaceutical products designed to combat obesity in the form of prescription drugs (anti-obesity drugs), over-the-counter substances such as tobacco, nutriceuticals, and supplements, and sweeteners and chemical fat-replacers on the market (such as olestra, approved for use in the United States).

North Americans also spend more than $33 billion on various weight-loss products, which may include both legitimate weight-loss services, exercise equipment, diet books, and pharmaceutical products, as well as questionable products or weight-loss "schemes." (Some experts estimate spending is closer to $50 billion when you add up the diet schemes sold on the Internet or on the black market.) By far, women dominate as consumers of diet books and exercise/weight-loss programs. Currently, roughly 80.4 per cent of Weight Watchers members are women, and women represent 70.7 per cent of all those using diet-control books; 63.7 per cent of those in exercise programs; and 59.2 per cent of those using meal supplements. Clearly, as discussed in Chapters 1 and 2, body image and cultural perceptions of "fat" – which do not match medical definitions of obesity – are at play. Indeed, many people purchasing diet-related products do not need them; the majority of consumers of diet products are not medically obese. Women of any size are able to obtain prescriptions for anti-obesity pills, as well as to purchase fraudulent diet pills frequently advertised as "fat burners" or "miracle pills." These products can be anything from food coloring, which works through the placebo effect, useless herbs, to even dangerous herbs, such as ephedra, which will be discussed later.

PRESCRIPTION DRUGS FOR WEIGHT LOSS

Drug treatment for obesity has a very shady history. Women in particular have been harmed by weight-loss drugs for many years. Throughout the 1950s, 1960s, and 1970s, women were routinely prescribed thyroxine, which is a thyroid hormone, to speed up their metabolisms. Unless a person has an underactive thyroid gland or no thyroid gland (which may have been surgically removed), this is a very dangerous medication that can cause heart failure. Request a thyroid-function test before you accept this medication. (For more information, see my book *The Thyroid Sourcebook*.)

Amphetamines or "speed" were also often widely prescribed to women by doctors, but they, too, can put your health at risk. One of the most notorious amphetamines (also called adrenergic stimulants), phentermine, still remains available, as does diethylpropion (Tenuate), phenmetrazine (Preludin), and mazindol. Both Health Canada and the Food and Drug Administration (FDA) recommend them for short-term use only, but people take these drugs for years; frequently they fill prescriptions and sell them to friends or acquaintances. Although some states in the United States have banned their prescription, people can simply purchase them in states where they are legal, on the street through various networks, or over the Internet. But amphetamines have serious side effects, including nervousness, insomnia, blood-pressure elevation, and mood change.

The basic problem with any prescription weight-loss drug, however, is that, as soon as the drug is stopped, weight is regained. Although obese people may lose 10 to 15 per cent of their initial body weight on diet pills, medication must be continued in order for this to be sustained. The side effects of all weight-loss drugs to date, however, make long-term use impossible, even life-threatening.

With the potential market that is waiting for an effective diet, it's logical to wonder why, with all of the technology and knowledge available to pharmaceutical companies, a good anti-obesity pill can't be developed. Obesity researchers have observed that creating an anti-obesity drug requires changing the human genetic code, which is designed to retain excess calories in preparation for famine. Our bodies were actually built to protect against weight loss rather than weight gain; this is how we survived and evolved throughout most of history, in which scarcity of food, rather than overabundance, was the danger.

The biological mechanisms in charge of our appetites and metabolism are much more complex than was once believed, and unfortunately they are not well understood. Drugs that attempt to change the way the biochemistry of our metabolism works end up disrupting too many systems at once. For example, appetite circuits in the brain use neurotransmitters and receptors that control other body processes. Anything designed to alter these sites cause terrible side effects, which have been the legacy of all the obesity pills to date. Developing an anti-obesity drug that is safe and effective for long-term – even lifetime – use is the challenge.

LESSONS LEARNED: A BRIEF HISTORY OF FEN-PHEN

One of the worst examples of the dangers of prescription weight-loss drugs can be seen in the fen-phen story. Trying to get "diet drugs" launched as a legitimate pharmaceutical product, Dr. Michael Weintraub and his colleagues at the University of Rochester published landmark studies in 1992 that urged the FDA to look upon Redux – the "fen" – as a treatment for the current obesity epidemic.

But Weintraub's studies had used a combination of phentermine (marketed as Ionamin, Fastin, and Adipex), an amphetamine that stimulated the adrenal system, in combination with fenfluramine (Pondimin), which increased serotonin release. While fenfluramine caused sedation, phentermine was stimulating. Weintraub studied the combination in several hundred patients for more than four years and found few side effects. The patients who lost weight on the combination regained less weight when compared to placebo controls. Furthermore, some people had a dramatic weight loss, while many patients reported that they stopped struggling with hunger and food obsessions on the combination. The two drugs were never approved for use by the FDA as a combo platter; prescribing them together was known as off-label prescribing, a common practice for many multiple drug therapies.

And thus, fenfluramine and phentermine became unofficially known as fen-phen. By 1996, a newer "fen" – dexfenfluramine (Redux) – was launched and became the standard "fen" prescribed with phen. It became the first new drug to promote weight loss approved by the FDA in more than twenty years.

In 1996, U.S. doctors wrote a total of 18 million monthly prescriptions for fen-phen. And many of the prescriptions were issued to people who were not obese. Some doctors even devoted their entire practices to fen-phen. Many physicians also lent their names to diets and products in exchange for a fee. Some doctors referred to themselves as a "bariatrician" (or "diet doctor"), which is not a board-certified specialty; in the United States, physicians simply sign up with the American Society of Bariatric Physicians.

In July 1997, the FDA and researchers at the Mayo Clinic and the Mayo Foundation made a joint announcement warning doctors that fen-phen can cause heart-valve problems. This was based on the report of twenty-four patients who had used fen-phen and now had heart-valve abnormalities. Since heart-valve problems are almost unheard of as a drug complication, no one normally looks for this in drug-trial testing. It was found by chance: a cardiac surgeon operating to replace a malfunctioning heart valve noted that it had a highly unusual appearance, which was only seen in patients who had a serotonin-producing tumor. High serotonin levels in fen-phen patients was found to be the culprit, and twenty-four cases of heart-valve damage in patients treated with fen-phen were discovered.

By August 28, 1997, the *New England Journal of Medicine* published five separate articles documenting new dangers associated with both fen-phen and Redux, including information from roughly a hundred cases of valvular abnormalities reported to the Centers for Disease Control. When almost three hundred patients were studied, about a third had abnormal heart valves. These heart-valve abnormalities involved a thickening of the valves on the left side of the heart, which could impair heart functioning, leading to fatigue, shortness of breath, fainting spells, chest pain, and swollen legs. On September 15, 1997, Redux and Pondimin were taken off the market.

In November 1997, the U.S. Department of Health and Human Services issued a warning, suggesting that anyone with exposure to either Pondimin or Redux be evaluated by a physician, with special attention to the presence of new heart murmurs. The fen-phen disaster ultimately cost Wyeth-Ayerst Laboratories $13.2 billion. The painful lesson not only underlined the unreliable studies with respect to "diet pills," but also reminded people of other situations in which women, in particular, have been harmed by therapies that were not properly tested prior to being put on the market.

NEW COMBO PLATTERS

With phentermine remaining on the market, researchers looked at other selective serotonin re-uptake inhibitors (SSRI) they could use with it. Fluoxetine (Prozac) seemed to have some effect on weight loss for the first four to six months, and seemed to help people with binge eating disorder; it also helped people with depression-related weight gain. Many weight-loss doctors now substituted Prozac for "fen" and continued to use phentermine. Yet the combination remains off-label prescribing, and has never been tested for efficacy or safety. Newer SSRIs, such as Bupropion (Wellbutrin or Zyban), became the more popular choice over Prozac, particularly for binge eaters. (It was also used with smokers as a smoking-cessation drug.) Bupropion, however, increases the incidence of seizures in bulimic patients. Other SSRIs such as fluoxetine (Prozac), sertraline (Zoloft), paroxetine (Paxil), or fluvoxamine (Luvox) continue to be prescribed with phentermine, without bad results so far.

MORE ANTI-OBESITY OFFERINGS

The two other anti-obesity drugs approved for use on the market are not that much safer than fen-phen. Orlistat (Xenical) blocks fat-digesting enzymes called lipases, preventing the digestion and absorption of fat. Each time you eat fat, you will therefore get rather embarrassing diarrhea that can be prevented by simply avoiding fat. But it hasn't worked out to be that simple. Orlistat also prevents the absorption of water molecules, and this, too, can cause cramping and severe diarrhea. The drug can also decrease absorption of vitamin D and other important nutrients.

Orlistat is the first drug to fight obesity through the intestine instead of the brain. Taken with each meal, it binds to certain pancreatic enzymes to block the digestion of 30 per cent of the fat you ingest. How it affects the pancreas in the long term is not known. Combined with a sensible diet, people on orlistat lost more weight than those not on orlistat. A review of orlistat trials found that the drug helped dieting patients lose an average of 2 to 3 per cent of their body weight as compared to diet alone. But people tended to gain the weight back after stopping orlistat. The sales of the drug are falling, because it is ineffective, with unacceptable side effects for some.

Sibutramine (Meridia, or Reductil in Europe) had promise when released in the 1990s; it was supposed to control appetite through neurotransmitters in the brain, having a similar function as Redux, which was pulled off the market in 1997. Side effects and deaths resulting from Meridia triggered a class-action lawsuit, an FDA investigation, and a withdrawal of the drug from Italian markets. Whenever neurotransmitters are involved, there are usually side effects, because they control so many other functions.

Between February 1998 and September 2001, 150 patients taking Meridia worldwide were hospitalized. Twenty-nine died – mostly from cardiovascular problems; the drug causes high blood pressure in particular, a side effect that was discovered in early clinical trials. In March 2002, consumer groups petitioned the FDA to withdraw the drug from the market. Abbot, which makes Meridia, responded to the petition by stating that the death rate from Meridia was far lower than that of any drug for the obese market. (In other words, high blood pressure is also inherently an obesity-related health complication.)

THE DASHED HOPES OF LEPTIN

The most promising anti-obesity treatment of all involved the "anti-fat hormone" leptin, which was first discovered in 1994 by a team of researchers at Rockefeller University in New York City and led to a surge of obesity-drug research. A mutant strain of extremely obese mice (lacking the gene to make leptin) were able to shed their weight when given leptin. On leptin, the mice's appetites decreased while their metabolic rates increased. Although it led researchers to hope that all obese people would lose weight on leptin, this did not occur. It turns out that, like the mutant obese mice, there are only a few rare cases of human obesity caused by leptin-deficiency. Everyone else becomes obese by eating too much and being too sedentary. The leptin discovery led to a successful treatment for rare and terribly sad cases of obesity in leptin-deficient individuals, however, who in the past would not have been able to lose weight.

HOW LEPTIN WORKS IN THE REST OF US

Most people who are obese actually have higher than normal blood levels of leptin, which is produced by fat cells, and are resistant to its actions. In leptin trials, the hormone was given to overweight people, and it was found that they were leptin-resistant because they had too much of it already. In fact, obesity researchers now believe that leptin has more to do with protecting against weight loss in times of famine than protecting against weight gain in times of plenty. When fat stores increase, so does leptin; when fat stores shrink, so does leptin. Appetite will increase and metabolism decreases when leptin levels shrink, but the opposite does not occur; appetite is not suppressed when leptin increases, nor is metabolism increased. Leptin, it seems, is one of those evolutionary hormones designed to keep our species alive, and protect us from starvation. Discovering leptin has led obesity researchers into finding out more about how appetite, fat stores, and "famine-protection" mechanisms work in the body.

ON THE HORIZON

In the wake of leptin research, a host of anti-obesity drugs are now in clinical trials. One drug causes the brain to produce Axokine, which works by activating a set of brain cells that produce appetite-dampening peptides. Again, because it works with brain chemistry, endocrinologists are skeptical about long-term effects. Drug research is also revolving around one hormone, ghrelin, which peaks before meals and triggers appetite, as well as a peptide that rises during meals and signals satiety. By stifling one and boosting the other, two more drugs could be developed for limiting calorie intake. Ghrelin is produced in the gastrointestinal tract; researchers describe it as "your stomach's way of telling your brain you're hungry." Drugs can be made to block ghrelin, which would kill hunger. Again, through calorie-intake reduction, such a drug could cause weight loss.

Perhaps one of the most exciting finds in obesity research, presented at the 2003 Endocrine Society meeting in Philadelphia, centers on the discovery of a brand-new hormone, known as PYY. While looking at the effects of bariatric surgery (stomach stapling) on appetite and the hormones secreted that make us feel full or satisfied, a British research team found that levels of the hormone

PYY surged in people who had undergone bariatric surgery. This research team suspects that PYY is responsible for a person's loss of the desire to eat excessively. Future research with PYY may lead to a truly effective obesity drug.

OVER-THE-COUNTER (OTC) WEIGHT-LOSS PRODUCTS

Weight-loss products, such as herbal formulations and supplements, are usually not reliable. However, one of the most successful OTC weight-loss products is not marketed as a "weight-loss" product, although it's been long known to suppress appetite – and shorten life span. It's called nicotine.

CIGARETTES

The chief reason women, in particular, start smoking is to suppress their appetites, a fact that has been well documented in tobacco studies and smoking-cessation research. The second most common ailment cigarettes "medicate" is stress, which often drives people to eat. So in a book about "fat," cigarettes fall into the category of a weight-loss product. Smoking satisfies "mouth hunger" – the need to have something in your mouth, which often occurs during stressful periods. It also slowly poisons your body, which is why it helps to suppress appetite. (Small daily doses of lethal poisons would have the same result.) The idea of controlling weight with cigarettes emerged in the 1920s when a tobacco-company wife was told by her doctor to smoke to "relax"; not only did smoking relax her, but it actually helped to curb her appetite. Thus the luring of women to cigarettes as a food replacement had begun. In fact, medical journals and the medical profession at that time actually recommended smoking to women as a way to "calm" them. Today, almost every woman who begins smoking does so for weight control. You've no doubt been bombarded with information about the health consequences of smoking. But many of you probably don't realize this alarming, yet underreported, fact: the number-one killer of women is cigarette smoking. Smoking-related diseases directly kill more women than any other health or social problem. Smoking-related diseases outnumber obesity-related diseases, and include lung cancer, heart disease, stroke, chronic lung disease, and other cancers more prevalent in smokers. All studies show that women who smoke "get sicker quicker." They develop, and die from, smoking-related diseases at much younger ages than men. It's not unusual for women in their thirties to develop lung cancer, for example. If you compare a man and a woman with similar smoking habits, the woman is twice as likely to die. Yet women are smoking in increasing numbers — almost always for weight control.

A single cigarette affects your body within seconds, increasing heart rate, blood pressure, and the demand for oxygen. The greater the demand for oxygen (because of constricted blood vessels and carbon monoxide, a by-product of cigarettes), the greater the risk of heart disease.

Tobacco companies use young women's body-image dilemmas as tools to addict them early to nicotine, which has devastating health consequences. Nonetheless, tobacco ads in women's magazines continue to sell the message to young women that smoking is "beautiful" or "glamorous."

Smoking began to be associated with "independence" in the 1960s, as the women's movement (also known as second-wave feminism) grew. By the late 1960s, one in three women in North America smoked. The popular Virginia Slims campaign slogan "You've Come a Long Way, Baby" played up the independence theme that seemed to attract women to cigarettes like moths to flame.

Tobacco companies continue to target women in their advertisements, especially aiming at international markets where rates of women smokers are much lower. They use Western "glamor" in their ads to entice women in developing countries to smoke —

women whose health risks are greater, due to extreme poverty and poor access to health care.

Without the awareness and decision-making powers of an informed adult, once a young girl buys into the marketing messages delivered to her by tobacco companies (e.g., smoking is glamorous, keeps you thin, etc.) and she begins smoking, she's hooked. Here's why: Nicotine produces a "controlled" response, enabling the smoker either to stimulate or calm herself. Small, shallow puffs on a cigarette enable a smoker to keep awake, alert, or active when she is fatigued. Deep drags from a cigarette give the smoker larger doses of nicotine, facilitating the release of endorphins, "feel good" chemicals the body makes naturally. Endorphins are released when we laugh, exercise, and do anything pleasurable, such as eating something tasty. Since the endorphins are coming from the body, smokers find that they do, in fact, perform better and are less stressed when they smoke more. On drugs such as amphetamines, heroine, or cocaine, the "high" is produced by the drug, not the body, so it feels completely different. Nicotine does not feel like a drug in the same way.

What is also addictive is the "control" the cigarette gives a person. Within seven to ten seconds of inhaling a cigarette, a concentrated dose of nicotine goes directly to the brain, producing a "rush," which in turn stimulates the release of a number of neurotransmitters, including dopamine and noradrenalin, a stress hormone. When a person tries to quit smoking, dopamine and noradrenalin levels drop, which produces a strong urge to smoke, in addition to withdrawal symptoms such as anxiety, depression, irritability, insomnia, difficulty concentrating, increased appetite, gastrointestinal discomfort, headaches, and lightheadedness. These withdrawal symptoms can actually worsen over a week, rather than lessen. The cravings can last for months. Most people begin to smoke again to relieve the suffering – especially during high periods of stress.

In the 1960s, when health warnings about smoking were issued, the tobacco industry introduced "light cigarettes" or "low-tar" cigarettes, which women bought in record numbers.

Women who wanted to quit smoking, or wanted to smoke without the health risks, bought the lie that a "lighter" cigarette is less harmful and "healthier." This is completely false. All cigarettes are made to deliver enough nicotine to keep you addicted. A light cigarette may be altered in that it smells differently, or appears less dense, but all research on light cigarettes since the 1980s have found that, when smokers switch to a light cigarette, they get the same dose of nicotine by taking deeper drags on the cigarette, and actually hold it in their lungs longer. In short, women who smoke light cigarettes wind up smoking *more* rather than less. More recent research has linked some forms of cancer to women who smoke light cigarettes.

WHY GIRLS START SMOKING
Studies show that eating disorders and smoking are intricately linked. In surveys young girls reveal that, when they are feeling "fat" or "ugly," they will smoke to cope with negative feelings about their bodies, and will substitute smoking for eating.

Young girls can turn to smoking when they begin to experience sexism or unfair situations that appear to favor men. The stresses of adolescence (body image, awakening sexuality, social awkwardness) can also lead them to smoking as a way of coping with growing up.

HERBAL CONCOCTIONS AND SUPPLEMENTS
Dieter's teas abound, as do many herbal supplements sold as a "natural way" to lose weight. Laci Le Beau Super Dieter's Tea, for example, contains mostly laxative properties such as senna, cascara sagrada, and diuretics. These products can cause diarrhea, cramping, and electrolyte imbalances. Many supplements and "diet teas" imported from China contain ephedra,

which is a Chinese stimulant similar to amphetamines. Phenyl-propanolamine, or PPA, is another stimulant found in many of these products.

EPHEDRA

Ephedra is a Chinese herb, known as desert herb, or *ma huang*. It grows in Mongolia and has been used in Chinese medicine for at least five thousand years. The substance ephedrine has been extracted from this herb and is used in both Western and Asian medicine as a decongestant and antihistamine to treat asthma, allergies, and sinus problems.

Ephedra also has a thermogenic effect, meaning that it increases basal metabolic rate, slightly raising body temperature and suppressing appetite, which causes calorie-burning in a way similar to any amphetamine (or speed). Just as amphetamines are notorious for heart-related problems, speeding up the heart rate, causing heart attacks, strokes, high blood pressure, and so forth, so is ephedra. When taken as directed, in very small amounts, ephedra is considered to be safe by many herbal practitioners and doctors who use the herb; but because it remains unregulated, few people take the amount as directed and often use it to get a "high" – particularly teens and twentysomethings. Ephedra is also routinely combined with many other substances, such as caffeine and illegal amphetamines.

Ephedra is sold in most health-food stores, and is used by millions of North Americans for weight loss. In 1999, two billion doses of ephedra were consumed, while ephedra-based supplements generated more than 900 million in sales for that year. Some knowingly purchase ephedra, while others are purchasing ephedra unknowingly; it is a common ingredient in special teas and in weight-loss supplements marketed under different names such as Ripped Fuel (for bodybuilders), Metabolife, and Diet-Phen (marketed to dieters). Caffeine is added either directly or indirectly; certain herbs that contain caffeine, such as guarana seeds or cola nuts, will be added to ephedra, giving the purchaser the perception that what s/he is buying is perfectly natural and safe because of so-called "natural" ingredients.

Because ephedra is a stimulant, when combined with other substances – especially caffeine, or a dangerous diet – it can lead to heart attacks, stroke, seizures, and death; it's also been linked to miscarriages in pregnant women who have taken it.

There is a difference between ephedrine alkaloids, which are present in the original herb, and the synthetic compound scientists derive from ephedra, known as ephedrine. Synthetic ephedrine, also found in various cold medications, can be easily identified on the label as "ephedrine hydrochloride." It is the synthetic ephedrine, which is considered to be the more potent version of ephedra, that is typically in weight-loss supplements.

In its April 5, 2001 issue, the *New England Journal of Medicine* published a review of ephedra, which analyzed records from 140 ephedra users who suffered complications between June 1997 and March 1999, finding about one-third of the problems definitely or probably were caused by the ephedra and another third possibly were caused by it. In one-fifth of the cases, there was insufficient information to draw conclusions, and the rest were deemed unrelated to ephedra use. The Ephedra Education Council, a group funded by supplement makers, counters that pre-existing health problems such as heart disease, not ephedra, caused the complications.

Many physicians stress that one must always consult a physician prior to taking ephedra. For example, it should not be taken by anyone who is pregnant or has a history of heart disease, stroke, psychiatric disorders, asthma, thyroid or kidney disease, diabetes, or prior seizures. That rules out a lot of people, yet many are unaware that they're taking ephedra because it's part of a supplement sold under a different name or label.

BANNING EPHEDRA

Although in the United States the supplement industry has exerted pressure on federal authorities seeking to ban ephedra or put warning labels on ephedra products, it remains available. In Canada, however, the product is being recalled. Health Canada requested in 2002 a recall from the market of certain products containing ephedra/ephedrine after a risk assessment concluded that these products pose a serious risk to health. This is a voluntary recall of products in which ephedra is likely a hidden ingredient in products marketed without FDA approval. The recall includes ephedra/ephedrine products having a dose unit of more than 8 mg of ephedrine or with a label recommending more than 8 mg/dose or 32 mg/day and/or are labeled or implied for use exceeding seven days, and of all combination products containing Ephedra/ephedrine, together with stimulants (e.g., caffeine) and other ingredients that might increase the effect of ephedra/ephedrine in the body. A full table of ingredients containing caffeine is attached to this advisory: ephedra/ephedrine products with labeled or implied claims for appetite suppression, weight-loss promotion, metabolic enhancement, increased exercise tolerance, body-building effects, euphoria, increased energy or wakefulness, or other stimulant effects. Health Canada also advises Canadians using ephedra to stop taking it. Currently, the maximum allowable dosages for ephedra/ephedrine in products is 8 mg ephedrine/single dose or 32 mg ephedrine/day. Products containing ephedra that are advised by physicians specifically will continue to be available, provided they do not contain caffeine and that the ephedrine content does not exceed 8 mg/dose to a maximum of 32 mg/day.

SAFER EPHEDRA

Herbal ephedra is sold in about two hundred unregulated dietary supplements, and past research has shown the dosage in ephedra pills often varies widely from what's on the label. It's estimated that roughly twelve million people used ephedra or ephedrine last year. According to the Ephedra Education Council, the following checklist can help you choose an authentic herbal ephedra that is actually the Chinese herb, *ma huang*.

- Avoid ephedra products that contain caffeine, which includes guarana and cola nuts.
- Avoid combining ephedra with any other over-the-counter or prescription drug you're taking.
- Discontinue use of ephedra if you experience any side effects at all.
- Never use ephedra if you have a health condition that affects your heart, such as high blood pressure, thyroid problems, or kidney problems.
- Never use ephedra if you're diabetic.
- Never use ephedra while pregnant or lactating.
- Never use ephedra for longer than one month.

FAKE "FAT-BURNER" DRUGS

Well, P.T. Barnum was right when he said, "There's a sucker born every minute." Otherwise these fat-burner peddlers would have melted away long ago. But they're out there in abundance!

"Fat burners" are not available over the counter, and are sold through e-mail spams, infomercials, and in advertorials alerting potential customers that a "new, miraculous" drug (which, of course, your doctor has never heard of) is in clinical trials now and literally melts away fat. These are not a bad scam, if you need to make a quick buck. They operate in a way similar to mortgage and loan scams. They get you to pay a fee for an evaluation, promise money in spite of your terrible credit ratings and high debt loads, and then reject your loan in spite of the "processing fee" you paid to be evaluated.

Here's what you do to market a fake diet pill: e-mail a million people and charge $50 for a six-month supply of the fake drug; hook in a thousand desperados who order it from your "secure server" with their credit card. If you're a real cad, you'll send them no product, and when the sucker tries to call or contact you, the phone will be disconnected and no trace will remain, since you close down your P.O. box. If you're nice, you'll send them some placebo capsules or fake pills, containing food coloring, sugar, and water or chitosan (see page 145). If you're truly in business, and want repeat orders, you'll send the suckers ephedrine, animal glandular tissue, and God knows what else. "Diet pills for kids," for example, is an ephedrine product. Health Canada and the FDA have been receiving increasing numbers of reports regarding the marketing of ephedrine, guarana, cola nut, white willow (salicin), and chromium as "fat burners," diet pills, or dietary supplements on the Internet. These products may also contain various amino acids and glandular products, some potentially toxic.

Fat-burner scammers usually collect the credit-card money in their merchant accounts, which are tied to some unnamed corporation. They fold up the bank account, close up shop, and e-mail again under a different address. Sounds like pretty easy money to me!

Be forewarned: If such a fat-burning drug truly existed, endocrinologists managing obese patients would know of it, and the top obesity researchers in the world would not be struggling with developing an effective, safe anti-obesity drug.

A CASE IN POINT

Many of the fake-fat-pill operators run advertorials in U.S. dailies – promising pills that burn fat. These usually consist of nothing more than direct-mail copywriting letters, purporting to be from medical doctors (no credentials or CVs are provided, of course). They are eager to share the information on their products that just melt your fat away. Claims about what the pills will do follow, stressing that they contain no chemical or drug and are perfectly natural. The doctors understand how fat and ugly you must feel, and point out how soon you can be thin; you are told that this is your golden opportunity to lose weight. There is no information about how the products work, or what they are. You're invited to order the drug by a 1-800 number or to mail back an order form to a legitimate address – often with a department number (likely a P.O. box number in disguise). People are often encouraged to help the companies with their research. They are asked to fill out a brief questionnaire, in which you agree to use the product for thirty days, and the company in question will send you a check for $50. You must provide personal information, including your name and telephone number.

What's wrong with this picture? First, the word *advertorial* on this sales pitch means that nothing in the ad can, or ought to, be taken seriously. Next, as a bioethicist, I can tell you that this is not how *ethical* researchers solicit human subjects for their research; it is in violation of every ethical code, including the new law in the United States, HIPAA (the Health Insurance Portability and Accountability Act).

Here's the skinny on these products. Many of them are actually a useless ingredient called chitosan, which is derived from chitin, a polysaccharide found in the exoskeleton of shellfish such as shrimp, lobster, and/or crabs. Many sellers claim that chitosan causes weight loss by binding fats in the stomach and preventing them from being digested and absorbed. There is no evidence that this product helps with weight loss; furthermore, since such minute quantities are provided to chitosan purchasers, it really does nothing. The British Advertising Standards Authority and the FDA have tried to crack down on chitosan pitches, fining various companies for breaching advertising and marketing standards. However, the advertisers claim that, since their advertisement was for a "food supplement," not a drug, they were not in breach of standards. The useless forms people fill out for some of these products are used to support the claim that the product works, in order to combat fines and lawsuits. All health authorities find this information to be unsubstantiated and the research meaningless. The two recent clinical trials on chitosan found it to be ineffective. People on placebos and on chitosan lost the same amount of weight: usually zero. Chitosan is not harmful, however; simply useless. Thus, companies can make money making weight-loss claims and promising safety for people of all health conditions, based on the theoretical uses of chitosan, without being accused of harming anyone. Taking people's money under false pretences, however, is still "harmful."

For the record, most products that claim to prevent fat absorption, "increase metabolism," "burn fat," or allow weight loss even if users eat high-fat foods are usually chitosan in a sleazy new ad. Others may be ephedrine in sleazy new ads too. For more information about diet-pill fraud, visit <www.quackwatch.com>, which frequently updates information about the latest scams.

FAT REPLACERS

In Chapter 4, I discussed the array of low-fat products, in light of a clarion call in 1990 for food manufacturers to speed up their development of more reduced-fat food choices. Thus, many foods were created from "fat replacers," which simulated many of the properties of fat in food, making it "creamy" or "smooth." Carbohydrate-based gums and starches, like guar gum and modified food starch, are common, including sugarlike compounds, fibers, and even fruit purees and applesauce. Carbohydrates can be used as thickeners, bulking agents, moisturizers, and stabilizers. For example, a new fat-replacing carbohydrate, oatrim (marketed by Golden Jersey Products under the brand name Replace), is an oat-flour ingredient added to some brands of skim milk in the United States. Oatrim contains a type of fiber called beta-glucan that may help lower blood cholesterol, in addition to providing fatlike creaminess. Unless they are new to the food supply, most carbohydrates-based fat replacers do not require government approval, because they are already in use and are safe. In the United States, this is termed Generally Recognized as Safe (GRAS). A few, including carrageenan (a seaweed derivative) and polydextrose, were submitted to the FDA for food-additive approval because they were new to the food supply, and were approved in April 2003.

Protein-based fat replacers are made from milk, whey, egg, soy, or other types of protein that have been manipulated to create appearance and what the industry calls "mouth feel" (which is texture and consistency).

Then there are fat-based fat replacers. Salatrim and caprenin are such fat replacers, and contain fatty acids that are partially but not completely digested, supplying five versus nine calories per gram. These fat replacers cannot be used to fry or sauté foods, but are used in products such as reduced-fat chocolate chips.

OLESTRA

The calorie-free fat substitute olestra is a fat-based fat replacer. It was approved for use in the United States by the FDA, and was developed by Procter and Gamble. But olestra is a potentially dangerous ingredient that most experts feel can do more harm than good. Canada has not yet approved it.

Olestra is known as a sucrose polyester made from a combination of vegetable oils and sugar. Therefore, it tastes just like the real thing, but the biochemical structure is a molecule too large for your liver to break down. So olestra gets passed into the large intestine and is excreted. Olestra is more than an "empty" molecule, however. It causes diarrhea and cramps and may deplete your body of vital nutrients, including vitamins A, D, E, and K, necessary for blood to clot. Some nutrition experts also fear a wider danger with olestra: instead of encouraging people to choose nutritious foods such as fruits, grains, and vegetables over high-fat foods, products like these encourage a high *fake*-fat diet that's still too low in fiber and other essential nutrients. And the no-fat icing on the cake is that these people could potentially wind up with a vitamin deficiency to boot.

Unlike other fat replacers, olestra is the only fat replacer that entirely replicates fat, including its use in frying, which is why it can be used in salty snacks. Olestra required FDA approval because it was a new food ingredient, not a combination of ingredients that were already in the food supply. A one-ounce portion of potato chips contains no fat when made with olestra and ten grams when made with oil.

Health Canada is taking the same stance as many nutrition experts, who find that the long-term consequences of olestra in the food supply haven't been addressed. Many experts feel it is tantamount to springing an untested chemical on the public. Even people who take supplements when using olestra will probably have the vitamins leached out of their intestine anyway.

The position of organizations such as the American Dietetic Association (ADA) is that fat-reduced or fat-replaced foods can only be part of a diet that includes plenty of fruits, vegetables, and grains (see Chapter 8). Fat replacers enable you to eat low-fat versions of familiar foods without making major changes in the way that you eat. But they should not be eaten in excess.

Critics of olestra argue that people will make the mistake of thinking "no fat" is healthy and choose olestra-containing Twinkies over fruits, trusting that they're eating well. Olestra is currently being used in snack foods only, but potential uses for olestra could include restaurant foods touted as "fat-free": fries, fried chicken, fish and chips, or onion rings. At home, olestra could be used as cooking oil for sautés, as a butter substitute for baking, or in a fat-free cheese. Potentially, we could be facing a future of eating "polyester foods." In fact, Procter and Gamble filed for olestra to be approved as a fat substitute for up to 35 per cent of the natural fats used in home cooking and up to 75 per cent of the fats used in commercial foods. It did not ask for approval to use olestra in table spreads or ice creams, however. When the FDA did not approve olestra for use in the products Procter and Gamble requested, a new request for olestra to be used only in salty snack foods was submitted. In 1996, the FDA approved olestra for use in savory snacks; Procter and Gamble proceeded to market the trade name for olestra, Olean. By 1998, Frito-Lay and Procter and Gamble announced the release of Olean products in dozens of snack foods, and the FDA approved this under the proviso that a warning label about olestra's health consequences be carried with each Olean product. (Current warnings about the product – for instance, when eaten in large amounts it can cause fecal leakage – are affixed to all

Olean products.) When the 1999 sales of Olean were disappointing, Procter and Gamble sought to have the warning removed; the FDA agreed to revise, but not remove, the label.

The Center for Science in the Public Interest has been opposed to the approval of olestra because of health concerns. In addition, studies have not found that olestra substantially reduces fat intake for the same reasons many low- or no-fat products have failed: people just eat more, a problem discussed in Chapter 1. Although olestra-made snacks taste identical to their originals, they still have plenty of calories from carbohydrates. People's behavior with olestra mirrors that of other low-fat snacks. They see olestra as a licence to eat more, rather than less and, ultimately, unless they practice the types of healthy-eating strategies discussed in Chapter 8, do not lose weight on olestra.

TYPES OF FAT REPLACERS

Carbohydrate-based fat replacers
- Maltodextrins. Baked goods.
- Starches. Baked goods, margarines, salad dressing, frozen desserts.
- Cellulose. Frozen desserts, sauces, salad dressings.
- Guar, xanthan, or other gums. Salad dressings.
- Polydextrose. Baked goods, cake mixes, puddings, frostings.
- Oatrim. Milk.

Protein-based fat replacers
- Protein concentrate (whey, egg white, soy). Frozen desserts, reduced-fat dairy products, and salad dressings.

Fat-based fat replacers
- Caprenin. Chocolate.
- Salatrim. Chocolate.
- Olestra (not in Canada). Snack chips, crackers.

SWEETENERS

Sweeteners were one of the first "fat pharm" foods that helped us to reduce caloric intake. A product can be sweet without containing a drop of sugar, thanks to the invention of artificial sugars and sweeteners. Artificial sweeteners will not affect your blood-sugar levels because they do not contain sugar; they may contain a tiny number of calories, however. It depends upon whether that sweetener is classified as nutritive or non-nutritive.

Nutritive sweeteners have calories or contain natural sugar. White or brown table sugar, molasses, honey, and syrup are all considered nutritive sweeteners. *Sugar alcohols* (see page 154) are also nutritive sweeteners, because they are made from fruits or produced commercially from dextrose. Sorbitol, mannitol, xylitol, and maltitol are all sugar alcohols. Sugar alcohols contain only four calories per gram, like ordinary sugar, and will affect your blood-sugar levels like ordinary sugar. It all depends on how much is consumed, and the degree of absorption from your digestive tract.

Non-nutritive sweeteners are sugar substitutes or artificial sweeteners; they do not have any calories and will not affect your blood-sugar levels. Examples of non-nutritive sweeteners are saccharin, cyclamate, aspartame, sucralose, and acesulfame potassium.

Table 7.1

Acceptable Daily Intake for Sweeteners

SWEETENER	INTAKE BASED ON MG/KG BODY WEIGHT
Aspartame	40
Ace-K	15
Cyclamate	11
Saccharin	5
Sucralose	9*

*Note: outside Canada, this figure reads 15.
Source: Canadian Diabetes Association, "Guidelines for the nutritional management of Diabetes Mellitus in the New Millenium. A Position Statement." Reprinted from *Canadian Journal Diabetes Care* 23 (3):56-69, 2000.

THE SWEETENER WARS

The oldest non-nutritive sweetener is saccharin, which is what you get when you purchase Sweet'N Low or Hermesetas. In Canada, saccharin can be used only as a tabletop sweetener in either tablet or powder form. Saccharin is three hundred times sweeter than sucrose (table sugar) but has a metallic aftertaste. At one point in the 1970s, saccharin was also thought to cause cancer, but this was never proven.

In the 1980s, aspartame was invented, and is now sold as NutraSweet. It was considered a nutritive sweetener because it was derived from natural sources (two amino acids, aspartic acid, and phenylalanine), which means that aspartame is digested and metabolized the same way as any other protein foods. For every gram of aspartame, there are four calories. But since aspartame is two hundred times sweeter than sugar, you don't need very much of it to achieve the desired sweetness. In at least ninety countries, aspartame is found in more than 150 product categories, including breakfast cereals, beverages, desserts, candy and gum, syrups, salad dressings, and various snack foods. Here's where it gets confusing: aspartame is also available as a tabletop sweetener under the brand name Equal and, most recently, PROSWEET. An interesting point about aspartame is that it's not recommended for baking or any other recipe where heat is required. The two amino acids in it separate with heat and the product loses its sweetness. That's not to say it's harmful if heated, but your recipe won't turn out.

For the moment, aspartame is considered safe for everybody, including people with diabetes, pregnant women, and children. The only people who are cautioned against consuming it are those with a rare hereditary disease known as phenylketonuria (PKU) because aspartame contains phenylalanine, which people with PKU cannot tolerate.

Another common tabletop sweetener is sucralose, sold as Splenda. Splenda is a white crystalline powder made from sugar. It's six hundred times sweeter than table sugar, but is not broken down in your digestive system, so has no calories at all. Splenda can also be used in hot or cold foods, and is found in hot and cold beverages, frozen foods, baked goods, and other packaged foods.

In the United States, you can still purchase cyclamate, a non-nutritive sweetener sold under the brand name Sucaryl or Sugar Twin. Cyclamate is also the sweetener used in many weight-control products and is thirty times sweeter than table sugar, with no aftertaste. Cyclamate is fine for hot or cold foods. In Canada, however, you can only find cyclamate as Sugar Twin or as a sugar substitute in medication.

The newest addition to the sweetener industry is acesulfame potassium (Ace-K), recently approved by Health Canada. About two hundred times sweeter than table sugar, Ace-K is sold as Sunett and is found in beverages, fruit spreads, baked goods, dessert bases, tabletop sweeteners, hard candies, chewing gum, and breath fresheners. While no specific studies on Ace-K and diabetes have been done, the only people who are cautioned against ingesting Ace-K are those on a potassium-restricted diet or people who are allergic to sulpha drugs.

Researchers at the University of Maryland have discovered another sweetener that can be specifically designed for people with diabetes. This sweetener would be based on D-tagatose, a hexose sugar found naturally in yogurt, cheese, or sterilized milk. The beauty of this ingredient is that D-tagatose has no effect on insulin levels or blood-sugar levels in people both with and without diabetes. Experts believe that D-tagatose is similar to acarbose in that it delays the absorption of carbohydrates.

D-tagatose looks identical to fructose, and has about 92 per cent of the sweetness of sucrose, except only 25 per cent of it will be metabolized. Currently, D-tagatose is being developed as a bulk sweetener. It is a few years away from being marketed and sold as a brand-name sweetener, however.

Stevia is a natural, non-fattening sweetener that is thirty to a hundred times sweeter than sugar, without any of the aftertaste that is common in many sugar substitutes. It is a herb that has been used in Paraguay and Brazil as a natural sweetener for centuries. It has been declared safe to use in Japan and is commonly found in soy sauce, chewing gum, and mouthwash. Stevia is high in chromium (a mineral that helps to regulate blood sugar); is a high source of manganese, potassium, selenium, silicon, sodium, and vitamin A; and contains iron, niacin, phosphorus, riboflavin, thiamine, vitamin C, and zinc.

There has been an explosion of interest in stevia because it is a natural alternative to sugar that contains many nutrients to boot. Stevia is not approved as a sweetener by the FDA; instead, it is legal only as a "dietary supplement." It also remains unapproved as a "food additive" in the United States. Stevia is available in Canada as a herbal product, but is not officially approved as a sweetener or food additive by Health Canada, Agrafood Canada, or the Canadian Diabetes Association.

Not to be confused with alcoholic beverages, sugar alcohols are nutritive sweeteners, like regular sugar. These are found naturally in fruits or are manufactured from carbohydrates. Sorbitol, mannitol, xylitol, maltitol, maltitol syrup, lactitol, isomalt, and hydrogenated starch hydrolysates are all sugar alcohols. In your body, these types of sugars are absorbed lower down in the digestive tract and will cause gastrointestinal symptoms if you use too much. Because sugar alcohols are absorbed more slowly, they were once touted as ideal for people with diabetes. But since they are a carbohydrate, they still increase your blood sugar – just like regular sugar. Now that artificial sweeteners are on the market in abundance, the only real advantage of sugar alcohols is that they don't cause cavities. The bacteria in your mouth doesn't like sugar alcohols as much as real sugar.

According to the FDA, even foods that contain sugar alcohols can be labeled "sugar-free." Sugar-alcohol products can also be labeled "Does not promote tooth decay," which is often confused with "low-calorie."

THE SKINNY

When it comes to anti-obesity drugs, long-term safety is always the problem, which is why we don't have any good anti-obesity drugs on the market; those that are on the market have many side effects or are legal amphetamines not intended for long-term use. A good anti-obesity drug should be safe to take for long periods of time in order to maintain weight loss; so far, no drugs can offer that. Studies show that most women will start smoking as a weight-loss method; in this case the harms associated with smoking-related diseases far outweigh the harms associated with obesity. Unsafe herbal supplements, which contain ephedrine and caffeine, as well as "fake drugs" abound; again, there are no good weight-loss products available over the counter. Many ephedrine-based products have been linked to adverse side effects and deaths. The one area where potentially useful products abound is in the area of fat and sugar replacers. Most consumer groups and nutritional experts warn that olestra is suspect, and for that reason has never been approved for use in Canada. Sweeteners are an alternative, particularly for families who want their children to kick the soft-drink habit. Allowing them to substitute the no-calorie version for their "liquid candy" (see Chapter 1) is a good start. Unfortunately, the best way to lose weight is the old-fashioned, sensible way; there is no weight-loss panacea on the pharmaceutical horizon yet.

CHAPTER 8

HEALTH, WELLNESS, AND THE
BALANCED DIET

No matter how many properties in foods are dissected or what kind of diet program you buy into, healthy eating and weight loss all come down to "balanced diet" – something that actually means a "balanced way of life." Again, the root word of diet – *diaita* – means "way of life."

Dietary guidelines from nutrition experts, government nutrition advisories and panels, and registered dieticians have not changed in fifty years. A good diet is *a balanced diet*, representing all food groups, based largely on plant-based foods such as fruits, vegetables, legumes, grains and grain products (collectively known as carbohydrates), with a balance of calories from animal-based foods such as meats (beef, poultry, etc.), fish, and dairy (also known as protein and fat). Nutrition research spanning the last fifty years has only confirmed these facts. What has changed in that time is the terminology used to define "good diet" and the bombardment of information we receive about which foods affect which physiological processes in the body, such as cholesterol levels or blood fats (a.k.a. triglycerides); blood-sugar levels (a.k.a. blood glucose or glycemic load); and insulin. There are also different kinds of "fats" and "carbohydrates," which has made eating so technical and scientific that ordinary North Americans feel more like chemists when trying to plan healthy meals and diets.

Big news and hoopla surround non-North American eating patterns, making the normal diets of other cultures, such as the French or Mediterranean or Asian diets, "nutrition news." These studies and news stories are often distorted. As we saw in Chapter 6, in the last ten years, a flurry of studies are looking at why, for example, olive oil and red wine would be healthy by dissecting their chemical compounds, and ignoring that people in those cultures also have a more balanced way of eating and living – which also may affect their health in positive ways.

Somehow we lost our balance when it comes to our diet. The food industry and the food lobby have encouraged us to eat more, rather than less. Food guidelines are also affected by the powerful food lobby. Dissecting the ingredients of food and telling us to stay away from "saturated fat," instead of real things we can relate to, such as beef, or cheese, or butter, reflects the food and agricultural industry's influence on government nutrition guidelines, which results in jargon.

That said, when you look at all the government food guidelines, and the sound diet programs, they all say the same thing: Eat largely plant-based foods, because they're low in calories but high in vitamins, minerals, fiber, and phytochemicals. Cut down on saturated fats (or foods of animal origin); use unsaturated or fish fats instead; and cut down on refined sugars. The most important component to any diet, however, is activity: using more energy (calories) than you ingest will maintain your body weight or lead to weight loss. This is what dieticians of the 1950s and 1960s called "a sensible" or "balanced diet." By 1990, it was called a low-fat diet. *But it's the same diet.*

THE OLD STORY OF LOW-FAT EATING

Original food guidelines and serving suggestions were designed in the early twentieth century to prevent malnutrition from vitamin deficiencies. By 1950, the problem of overnutrition began to be evident. In her book *Food Politics*, Marion Nestle presents dietary guidelines from a 1959 book on heart disease, *Eat Well and Stay Well*, which was written by physician Ancel Keys and his wife, Margaret Keys. The guidelines for a "healthy heart" at that time were almost identical to today's dietary guidelines: maintaining normal body weight; restricting saturated fats and red meat; using polyunsaturated fats instead to a maximum of 30 per cent of daily calories; plenty of fresh fruits and vegetables and non-fat milk products; avoidance of overly salted foods and refined sugar. The Keyses' guidelines even recommended getting exercise, stopping smoking, and reducing stress!

In the early 1960s, the American Heart Association, based on its research from the mid-1950s, issued almost identical guidelines, with these small changes: reducing fat intake to a maximum of 35 per cent of daily calories, with saturated fats reduced to 10 per cent of calories, and cholesterol restricted to 300 mg.

From 1958 to 1990, the United States's federal guidelines on meat consumption did not change, even though the wording did. For example, in 1958, four to six ounces, or two servings of meat per day, were recommended, which was far less than other food-group servings. In the 1970s, the recommendations were to "decrease fatty meat," and in 1979, the serving size was still four to six ounces, or two servings. By the 1980s, the recommendations were to "choose lean meats."

Then by 1990, as active living was virtually engineered out of most people's lives, and people became more conscious about the problem with red meat, the beef lobby began to influence the guidelines, which were raised to "2 to 3 servings, or 6 ounces of meat," which encouraged people to eat more meat than in the past. In 1992, "2 to 3 servings of lean meat" was recommended, with 5 to 7 ounces as a serving size. By 1995, it got more specific: "choose 2 to 3 servings of lean meats (4 to 9 ounces!) and limit intake of high-fat processed meats, and limit intake of organ meats." By 2000, the guidelines were the same as 1995, with additional limitations of liver and other organ meats and use of animal fats. When people started getting fatter (the real obesity explosion occurred in the mid-1990s), the diet books flew off the shelves; but all of the sound diet books echoed the very same advice we find in the Keyses' 1959 book. Sensible diets, in other words, have not changed; the people controlling our diets have. And that is the food industry, not the government.

As discussed in Chapter 1, most people's diets do not even come close to balanced. Many North Americans eat nothing *but* the types of foods that have always been discouraged: saturated fats (thanks to fast food), sugar (thanks to the soft-drink industry), refined carbohydrates (thanks to snack foods), and not enough fiber.

Again, losing weight means eating fewer calories and/or expending more calories than you eat. Fat has more calories per gram than carbohydrates (nine versus four calories per gram). Saturated fats are the building blocks of clogged arteries and cardiovascular problems; unsaturated fats are heart-protective. We can therefore choose the right type of fat over the wrong type of fat. But overall, weight loss, *by simply eating less*, will have more of an impact on reducing obesity and obesity-related health problems than "splitting fats" at the end of the day.

ALL BALANCED DIETS *ARE* LOW-FAT DIETS

With the exception of low-carb diets, which ultimately are still low-calorie diets (see Chapter 5), any balanced diet that is rated acceptable by board-certified dieticians, nutritionists, or consumer watchdog organizations, such as the Centre for Science in the Public Interest, will be what is called a "low-fat" diet by today's standards. One of the best kept secrets, in fact, is the Canadian Diabetes Association's dietary guidelines (the American Diabetes

Association has a different system, but similar guidelines). Anyone following the diabetes association guidelines from any country will be eating well-balanced, low-fat meals. The diets discussed in Chapter 4, however, are *very low-fat diets*, recommended only for people who need to reverse heart disease quickly, and are not recommended for the masses – or for people with type 2 diabetes without consulting a certified diabetes educator.

Programs such as Weight Watchers or Jenny Craig, or similar programs by brand-name weight-loss centers, emphasize calorie reduction through different techniques. Even weight-loss "replacement meal shakes" do just that. The technique you like is the one that will probably work best for you.

The most popular program by its success rate, based on long-term sustainability and maintenance, is Weight Watchers, which is pure calorie-counting. The disadvantage to calorie counting is that a chocolate bar may contain the same calories/points as a large sandwich, but it's not as healthy or nutritious (although dark chocolate has now been found to carry some heart-health benefits). Nonetheless, by being aware of the calories, most people ultimately use their Weight Watchers points more judiciously and the point system allows people some leverage for indulging without feeling that they "blew" their diets. Discouragement from dieting is what the Weight Watchers system helps to offset.

Programs like Jenny Craig are similar, but make most of their money from getting you to buy their brand of low-calorie packaged foods or meals; all of their meal plans are based on meals that use their foods. But these weight-loss organizations have some added support group/motivational seminars or classes, weigh-ins to keep you focused and goal-oriented, and, most important, education about how to shop in today's confusing world of labels and overabundance of fast foods and restaurants and behavioral counseling about eating habits. The added support in addition to the diet can be beneficial, particularly to women, who generally like to share experiences. People who dislike discussion groups will probably not like Weight Watchers-like programs, but there are also online versions of many of these programs. People are usually charged for missing classes (which run about $10 to $15 per class). Classes are emphasized to make it clear that eating behavior is just as important as the diet itself.

Ultimately, most people, regardless of the weight-loss program chosen, will probably wind up with a diet that is balanced, looking something like 40 per cent carbs, 30 per cent protein, and 30 per cent fat.

Some diets call themselves "low carb" or "high protein" (see Chapter 5) but are balanced low-fat diets too. One example is the Zone, which was found to be too low in whole grains and calcium by the Center for Science in the Public Interest but otherwise fairly balanced. Any diet that limits calories, not entire food groups, is just fine. For example, a vegetarian diet may eliminate "meats," but not "fats" – which is a food group. Pick one you like and fly with it. You can judge a good diet based on these four questions:

1. Are all food groups included: plant-based (fruits and vegetables); grains and complex carbs; proteins (lean meats); fats? If not, stay away.

2. Are you encouraged to have *the least* number of calories from fats, and discouraged from junk foods and refined sugars? If so, this is sensible.

3. Does the weight loss promised average about one to two pounds per week, or is weight loss of ten or more pounds per week promised? Anything more than one to two pounds a week is suspicious and likely "faddish." Gradual weight loss is sustainable for life; speedy weight loss leads to yo-yo effects, where you gain as much back as you lost.

4. Is it a diet that offers enough variety that you would feel good eating this way for life, and feeding your whole family with the foods encouraged? People on the Atkins diet, for example (see Chapter 5), have stated that they "can't take it" beyond a certain point, and cannot feed their children with the diet.

RAPID WEIGHT-LOSS DIETS

Any diet that causes you to lose weight rapidly (such as five to ten pounds per week) in the absence of activity is not a diet you'll be able to sustain for the long term. Even people who lose weight rapidly due to illness or depression (which frequently results in a ten-pound weight loss) will regain their weight once they regain their health. Liquid diets, starvation diets, or taking weight-loss herbs or drugs that suppress your appetite (see Chapter 7) may lead to significant weight loss that will make you feel "high" in the short term, but will not provide you with a practical, sensible, nutritious diet for life. The motivation you can gain from seeing "quick results" may lead some people to seek out a "maintenance" diet such as Weight Watchers, in order to stay at their desired weight, but most people will find it difficult to resume normal eating habits and keep their weight off at the same time. The body adapts to rapid weight loss by going into "surviving the famine" mode, whereby it becomes more efficient at using calories and storing fat. Starvation or rapid-weight-loss diets will simply cause the body to store calories as fat more efficiently than before "the diet." Many obese people have said that they "dieted" up to the weights they are at.

Some low-calorie diets advertise that you can "eat all the fat you want and lose weight." The Atkins diet is a good example. After a more careful analysis (see Chapter 5), we have seen that the Atkins diet is a low-calorie diet of about 1,200 to 1,500 calories per day; it works because of compliance and motivation. People stick to the diet because the food is more appealing to them; they're motivated to stay on it because they lose double the weight as on ordinary diets. But, ultimately, the diet makes people feel unwell, and most become tired of being deprived of so many crucial nutrients. Thus, it is a short-term diet that is not sustainable. The weight loss is due to eating fewer calories, and inducing a "survival" mechanism in the body that will suppress appetite as it would in times of famine. Starving yourself will do the same thing; but is this a way to live?

THE COMPONENTS OF A BALANCED DIET

Let's examine the components of a balanced diet. Carbohydrates are the main source of fuel for muscles. Protein is the "cell food" that helps cells grow and repair themselves. Fat is a crucial nutrient that can be burned as an alternative fuel in times of hunger or famine. Simple sugars that do not contain any fat will convert quickly into energy or be stored as fat.

Your body will change carbohydrates into glucose for energy. If you eat more carbohydrates than you can burn, your body will turn the extra into fat. The protein your body makes comes from the protein you eat. As for fats, they are not broken down into glucose, and are usually stored as fat. The main problem with fatty foods is that they have double the calories per gram compared with carbohydrates and protein. This results in your gaining weight. Too much saturated fat, as discussed throughout this book, can increase your risk of developing cardiovascular problems. What we also know is that the rate at which glucose is absorbed by your body from starch and sugars is affected by other parts of your meal, such as the protein, fiber, and fat. If you're eating only carbohydrates and no protein or fat, for example, your blood sugar will go up faster, which is why people can gain weight when they don't eat properly on a low-fat diet.

The best advice is to limit carbohydrates in each meal to about 40 per cent, and be sure to have about 30 per cent protein and 30 per cent of "helpful" fat. Canadian nutrition guidelines stipulate that your daily intake of protein (animal products) shouldn't exceed 20 per cent (British guidelines stipulate 15 per cent). The American Diabetes Association guidelines state that a healthy diet should consist mainly of complex carbohydrates (roughly 50 per cent) with about 30 per cent of your energy from fat – and less than 10 per cent from saturated fats. The exact composition may vary, but you're aiming for mostly complex, or "good," carbs (fruits, veggies, and grains) and, minimally, saturated fats or "bad fats" and refined sugar ("bad carbs"). Balance the rest.

Today's balanced, healthy diets encourage you to:

1. Maximize GOOD CARBS, minimize BAD FATS.
    Good carbs include vegetables, fruit, potatoes, whole-wheat bread, pasta, rice, oats, beans, soy, and whole-grain cereals. Bad fats are foods that are highly saturated, such as cheeseburgers, milkshakes, butter, and fatty dairy products or foods that have trans fatty acids, such as anything hydrogenated.

2. Maximize GOOD FATS, minimize BAD CARBS.
    Good fats include monounsaturated or polyunsaturated fats, such as olive oil or omega-3 and omega-6 fatty acids, which are found in fish swimming in cold waters (e.g., salmon, sardines). Bad carbs are high in starch and refined sugar, such as crackers, cookies, cakes, and potato chips.

3. Minimize TOTAL FATS.
    Limit total calories from fat to about 20 per cent to 30 per cent. Good or bad, fat contains more than twice the calories of other foods and should be eaten in reduced quantities if you want to lose weight.

UNDERSTANDING FAT

Fat is technically known as fatty acids, which are crucial nutrients for our cells. We cannot live without fatty acids. If you looked at each fat molecule carefully, you'd find three different kinds of fatty acids on it: saturated (solid), monounsaturated (less solid, with the exception of olive and peanut oils), and polyunsaturated (liquid) fatty acids. (When you see the term *unsaturated fat*, this refers to either monounsaturated or polyunsaturated fats.)

These three fatty acids combine with glycerol to make what's chemically known as triglycerides. Each fat molecule is a link chain made up of glycerol, carbon atoms, and hydrogen atoms.

The more hydrogen atoms that are on that chain, the more saturated or solid the fat. The liver breaks down fat molecules by secreting bile, stored in the gallbladder (this is its sole function). The liver also makes cholesterol. Too much saturated fat may cause your liver to overproduce cholesterol, while the triglycerides in your bloodstream will rise, perpetuating the problem.

Fat is a good thing in moderation. But like all good things, most of us want too much of it. Excess dietary fat is by far the most damaging element in the Western diet. A gram of dietary fat contains twice the calories as the same amount of protein or carbohydrate. Fat in the diet comes from meats, dairy products, and vegetable oils. Other sources of fat include coconuts (60 per cent fat), peanuts (78 per cent fat), and avocados (82 per cent fat).

To cut through all this big fat jargon, you can boil down fat into two categories: "harmful fats" and "helpful fats," which the popular press often defines as "good fats" and "bad fats."

HARMFUL FATS

The following are harmful fats because they can increase your risk of cardiovascular problems, as well as many cancers, including colon and breast cancers. These are fats that are fine in moderation, but harmful in excess (and harmless if not eaten at all):

- Saturated fats. These are solid at room temperature and stimulate cholesterol production in your body when the liver has to work hard to break them down. The way that saturated fat looks prior to ingesting it is the way cholesterol will look when it lines your arteries. Foods high in saturated fat include processed meat, fatty meat, lard, butter, solid vegetable shortening, chocolate, and tropical oils (coconut oil is more than 90 per cent saturated). Saturated fat should be consumed only in very low amounts.
- Trans fatty acids. These are factory-made fats that behave just like saturated fat in your body; they're often found in margarine.

HELPFUL FATS

Helpful fats are beneficial to your health and protect against certain health problems. You are encouraged to use more, rather than less, of these fats in your diet. In fact, nutritionists suggest that you substitute these for harmful fats:

- Unsaturated fats. This kind of fat is partially solid or liquid at room temperature. The more liquid the fat, the more unsaturated it is, which lowers your cholesterol levels. This group of fats includes monounsaturated fats and polyunsaturated fats. Sources of unsaturated fats include vegetable oils (canola, safflower, sunflower, corn, olive) and seeds and nuts. Unsaturated fats come from plants, with the exception of tropical oils, such as coconut, which are saturated.
- Fish fats (a.k.a. omega-3 fatty acids). The fats naturally present in fish that swim in cold waters, known as omega-3 fatty acids or fish oils, are all polyunsaturated. Again, polyunsaturated fats are good for you: they lower cholesterol levels, are crucial for brain tissue, and protect against heart disease. Include cold-water fish like mackerel, albacore tuna, salmon, and sardines in your diet.

FACTORY-MADE FATS

An assortment of factory-made fats have been introduced into our diet, courtesy of food producers who are trying to give us the taste of fat without all the calories of saturated fats. Unfortunately, manufactured fats offer their own bag of horrors. That's because, when a fat is made in a factory, it becomes a trans fatty acid, a harmful fat that not only raises the level of "bad" cholesterol (LDL) in your bloodstream but also lowers the amount of "good" cholesterol (HDL) that's already there.

How, exactly, does a trans fatty acid come into being? Trans fatty acids are what you get when you make a liquid oil, such as corn oil, into a more solid or spreadable substance, such as margarine. Trans fatty acids, you might say, are the road to hell, paved with good intentions. Someone way back when thought that if you could take the "good fat" – unsaturated fat – and solidify it so it could double as butter or lard, you could eat the same things without missing the spreadable fat. That sounds like a great idea. Unfortunately, to make an unsaturated liquid fat more solid, hydrogen is added to its molecules. This process, known as *hydrogenation*, converts liquid fat to semi-solid fat. That ever-popular chocolate-bar ingredient "hydrogenated palm oil" is a classic example of a trans fatty acid. Hydrogenation also prolongs the shelf life of a fat, such as polyunsaturated fats, which can oxidize when exposed to air, causing rancid odors or flavors. Deep-frying oils used in the restaurant trade are generally hydrogenated.

Trans fatty acid is sold as a polyunsaturated or mono-unsaturated fat with a label that reads: "Made from polyunsaturated vegetable oil." There's one problem. In your body, it is treated as a saturated fat. So, really, trans fatty acids are a saturated fat in disguise. The advertiser may, in fact, say that the product contains "no saturated fat" or is "healthier" than the comparable animal- or tropical-oil product with saturated fat. So be careful out there: read your labels. The key word you're looking for is *hydrogenated*. If the product lists a variety of unsaturated fats (monounsaturated X oil, polyunsaturated Y oil), keep reading. If the word *hydrogenated* appears, count that product as a saturated fat; your body will!

Since the news of trans fatty acids broke in the late 1980s, margarine manufacturers have begun offering some less-harmful margarines; some contain no hydrogenated oils, while others contain much smaller amounts. Margarines with less than 60 to 80 per cent oil (9 to 11 grams of fat) will contain 1 to 3 grams of trans fatty acids per serving, compared to butter, which is 53 per cent saturated fat. You might say it's a choice between a bad fat and a worse fat.

It's also possible for a liquid vegetable oil to retain a high concentration of unsaturated fat when it's been partially hydrogenated. In this case, your body will metabolize this as some saturated fat and some unsaturated fat.

Recommendations for Fat

TYPE OF FAT	HOW MUCH TO EAT
Total fat requirements	no more than 30 per cent of daily energy
Saturated and polyunsaturated fat requirements	no more than 10 per cent of daily energy
Monounsaturated fat	as much as possible
Fish fat	a serving at least once a week
Trans fatty acids	limit as much as possible

Source: Canadian Diabetes Association, "Guidelines for the nutritional management of Diabetes Mellitus in the New Millennium. A Position Statement." Reprinted from *Canadian Journal Diabetes Care* 23 (3):56-69, 2000.

UNDERSTANDING CARBOHYDRATES

A diet high in carbohydrates can also make you fat, because excess carbohydrates (starchy stuff such as rice, pasta, breads, or potatoes) are stored as fat. Carbohydrates can be simple or complex. Simple carbohydrates are found in any food that contains natural sugar (honey, fruits, juices, vegetables, milk) and anything that contains table sugar. Complex carbohydrates are more sophisticated foods that are made up of larger molecules, such as grain foods, starches, and foods high in fiber.

Normally, all carbs convert into glucose when you eat them. Glucose is the technical term for "simplest sugar." All your energy comes from the glucose in your blood, also known as blood glucose or blood sugar. When your blood sugar is used up, you feel weak, tired, and hungry. But what happens when you eat more carbohydrates than your body can use? Your body stores those extra carbs as fat. What we also know is that the rate at which glucose is absorbed by your body from carbohydrates is affected by other parts of your meal, such as the protein, fiber, and fat you consume. If you're eating only carbohydrates and no protein or fat, for example, they will convert into glucose more quickly, to the point where you may experience mood swings as your blood sugar rises and dips.

FIBER: A GOOD CARB

If you look at the box on page 163, the first building block for a healthy diet is to: maximize GOOD CARBS and minimize BAD FATS. The best way to do this is to incorporate fiber into your diet. Fiber is the quintessential "good carb"; you can ingest both water-soluble fiber (which dissolves in water) and water-insoluble fiber (which does not dissolve in water but, instead, absorbs water). While soluble and insoluble fiber do differ, they are equally beneficial. It is the insoluble fiber that promotes regularity, meaning it prevents constipation, which also is a crucial component in preventing colon cancer. Fiber also takes much longer to digest, which keeps you feeling less hungry, and keeps your blood-sugar levels more stable. This will help you eat less!

As the insoluble fiber moves through the digestive tract, it absorbs water like a sponge and helps to form waste into a solid form faster, making the stools larger, softer, and easier to pass. Without insoluble fiber, solid waste gets pushed down to the colon or lower intestine as always, where it is stored and dried out until you're ready to have a bowel movement. This is exacerbated when you ignore the urge, as the colon further dehydrates the waste until it becomes harder and difficult to pass, a condition known as constipation.

In other words, insoluble fiber increases the transit time by increasing colon motility and limiting the length of time dietary toxins hang around the intestinal wall. This is why it can dramatically decrease your risk of colon cancer.

Good sources of insoluble fiber are skins from various fruits and vegetables, seeds, leafy greens and cruciferous vegetables (cauliflower, broccoli, Brussels sprouts), and wheat bran and whole grains. The problem is understanding what is truly "whole grain." There is an assumption that because bread is dark or brown, it's more nutritious; this isn't so. In fact, many brown breads are simply enriched white breads dyed with molasses. ("Enriched" means that nutrients lost during processing have been replaced.) High-fiber pita breads and bagels are available, but you have to search for them. A good rule is to look for the phrase *whole wheat* on the product label, which means that the wheat is, indeed, whole.

Soluble fiber lowers the bad cholesterol (LDL) in your body. Experts aren't entirely sure how soluble fiber works, but one popular theory is that it gets mixed into the bile the liver secretes and forms a type of gel that traps the building blocks of cholesterol, thus lowering harmful LDL levels. This action is akin to a spiderweb trapping smaller insects.

Good sources of soluble fiber include oats or oat bran, legumes (dried beans and peas), some seeds, carrots, oranges, bananas, and other fruits. Soybeans are also high in soluble fiber. Studies show that people with very high cholesterol have the most to gain by eating soybeans. Soybean is also a phytoestrogen that is believed to lower the risks of estrogen-dependent cancers, as well as lower the incidence of estrogen-loss symptoms associated with menopause.

WHAT'S IN A GRAIN?

For thousands of years, cooked whole grains were the dietary staple for all cultures. Rice and millet in the Orient; wheat, oats, and rye in Europe; buckwheat in Russia; sorghum in Africa; barley in the Middle East; and corn in pre-European North America.

Most of us turn to grains and cereals to boost our fiber intake, which experts recommend should be at about 25 to 35 grams per day. Use the chart on page 171 to help gauge whether you're getting enough. The list measures the amount of insoluble fiber. An easy way to boost your fiber intake is to add pure wheat bran to your foods. It is available in health food stores or supermarkets in a sort of "sawdust" form. Three tablespoons of wheat bran is equal to 4.4 grams of fiber. Sprinkle one to two tablespoons onto cereals, rice, pasta, or meat dishes. You can also sprinkle it into orange juice or low-fat yogurt. It has virtually no calories. It's important to drink a glass of water with your wheat bran, as well as a glass of water after you've finished your wheat-bran-enriched meal.

WATER AND FIBER

How many people do you know who say, "But I do eat tons of fiber and I'm still constipated!" Probably quite a few. The reason they remain constipated in spite of their high-fiber diet is that they are not drinking water with it. It is important to note that water means water. Milk, coffee, tea, soft drinks, or juice are not a substitute for water. Unless you drink water with your fiber, the fiber will not bulk up in your colon to create the nice, soft bowel movements you desire. Again, think of fiber as a sponge. You must soak a dry sponge with water in order for it to be useful. Same thing here. Fiber without water is as useful as a dry sponge. *You gotta soak your fiber!* So here is the fiber/water recipe:

- Drink three glasses of water with your fiber. This means having a glass of water with whatever you're eating. Even if what you're eating does not contain much fiber, drinking water with your meal is a good habit to get into.
- Drink two glasses of water after you eat.

There are, of course, other reasons to drink lots of water throughout the day. For example, some studies show that dehydration can lead to mood swings and depression. Women are often advised by numerous health and beauty experts to drink eight to ten glasses of water per day for other reasons: water helps you to lose weight and to have well-hydrated, beautiful skin; it also helps you to urinate regularly, important for bladder function (women, in particular, suffer from bladder infections and urinary incontinence). By drinking water with your fiber, you'll be able to get up to that eight glasses of water per day in no time.

The Fiber Chart

CEREALS	GRAMS OF FIBER
(based on 1/2 cup unless otherwise specified)	
Fiber First Multibran	15.0
Fiber One	12.8
All-Bran	10.0
Oatmeal (1 cup)	5.0
Raisin Bran (3/4 cup)	4.6
Bran Flakes (1 cup)	4.4
Shreddies (2/3 cup)	2.7
Cheerios (1 cup)	2.2
Corn Flakes (1.5 cups)	0.8
Special K (1.5 cup)	0.4
Rice Krispies (1.5 cup)	0.3

BREADS	GRAMS OF FIBER
(based on 1 slice)	
Rye	2.0
Pumpernickel	2.0
Twelve grain	1.7
100% whole wheat	1.3
Raisin	1.0
Cracked wheat	1.0
White	0

Keep in mind that some of the newer high-fiber breads on the market today have up to seven grams of fiber per slice. This chart is based on what is normally found in typical grocery stores.

FRUITS AND VEGGIES

Another easy way of boosting fiber content is to know how much fiber your fruits and vegetables pack per serving. All fruits, beans (a.k.a. legumes), and vegetables listed here show measurements for insoluble fiber, which is not only good for colon health but for your heart. Some of these numbers may surprise you!

FRUIT	GRAMS OF FIBER
Raspberries (3/4 cup)	6.4
Strawberries (1 cup)	4.0
Blackberries (1/2 cup)	3.9
Orange (1)	3.0
Apple (1)	2.0
Pear (1/2 medium)	2.0
Grapefruit (1/2 cup)	1.1
Kiwi (1)	1.0

BEANS	GRAMS OF FIBER
(based on 1/2 cup unless otherwise specified)	
Green beans (1 cup)	4.0
White beans	3.6
Kidney beans	3.3
Pinto beans	3.3
Lima beans	3.2

VEGETABLES	GRAMS OF FIBER
(based on 1/2 cup unless otherwise specified)	
Baked potato with skin (1 large)	4.0
Acorn squash	3.8
Peas	3.0
Creamed, canned corn	2.7
Brussels sprouts	2.3
Asparagus (3/4 cup)	2.3
Corn kernels	2.1
Zucchini	1.4
Carrots (cooked)	1.2
Broccoli	1.1

WHO CAN HELP US EAT BETTER?

Knowing all this information is not going to help you eat well if you don't have access to a healthy, high-quality food supply or food labels you can read and understand. When we think about who protects our diet we may look to departments or ministries of health, food, water, agriculture, finance, education, industry, social services, and trade. But that is not who is ultimately in charge. Food companies have a tremendous influence on creating food policies, guidelines, and labeling. For example, food companies sponsor the educational activities of nutritional professional societies, as well as the work of individual scientists researching diet and nutrition.

Food companies are often the only source of funding for researchers; by the mid-1970s, it was commonplace for food companies to offer honoraria to academic faculty in agriculture and nutrition for consulting services on advisory boards, lecturing at conferences, and so on. Food companies sponsor almost every aspect of nutrition research published in peer-reviewed journals, as well as the production of entire journals and supplements. One of the most frequent sponsors includes Coca-Cola, for example. These sponsors even frequently influence what gets researched. Remember the Mediterranean diet discussed in Chapter 6? Much of the research on olive oil and the Mediterranean diet is sponsored by the International Olive Oil Council. A recent study (2000) on chocolate, extolling its heart-healthy virtues, was sponsored by a cocoa council and a chocolate-bar company. And on it goes. A typical academic nutrition conference may include a Kellogg's sponsored breakfast, which features a panel debating the latest fiber research, lunch supplied by a dairy organization with cheesy dairy treats, and a panel on the latest in calcium research. Then the conference may move on to a fancy dinner, sponsored by a beef organization, where wonderful prime rib is served, and a talk about "new thinking about beef" is delivered. Vitamin manufacturers may push the idea of fortifying foods with various vitamins. Many children's cereals are nothing short of sugar and vitamins – but advertising tells children that they're nutritious.

Food companies all have particular agendas in pushing nutritional guidelines and standards in their favor. When you read in the paper, for example, that "high-fiber cereals may reduce the risk of some cancers," you can bet that a cereal company is behind that study. Studies concluding that it's okay to eat eggs, because there was "no increase in study participants' cholesterol readings" may have been sponsored by an egg-marketing board. On it goes. Margarine studies may be sponsored by margarine companies; lactose-intolerance studies, showing how lactose intolerance is "not that prevalent," may be sponsored by dairy companies. Wine studies are sponsored by wine makers or wine councils. Sodium studies (which concluded that there's no relationship between sodium and high blood pressure, of course) are sponsored by Campbell's. Dietary guidelines and labels have become subtle advertisements for food companies. Health claims on labels have become routine, which serves to confuse, more than guide, us in our choices.

In the United States, Heinz tried to use its influence to get ketchup labels to read that the food could reduce cervical and prostate cancer, based on studies showing that the phytochemical lycopene could be a factor in protecting against it. Not only is this not conclusive, but since Heinz ketchup is a condiment, containing a lot sugar and salt, it is stretching it to say that a dab of ketchup would carry any health benefit. In 1999, Heinz ran an ad in the *New York Times*, making the claim that "lycopene may help reduce the risk of prostate and cervical cancer," with a bold picture of Heinz ketchup, and a reference to a journal article linking lycopene to a possible reduction in these cancers (see Chapter 3). It also featured an endorsement from the Cancer Research Foundation of America. The ad was eventually pulled. The Heinz case, however, demonstrates that you can't believe everything you read on a label.

GETTING THE FOOD INDUSTRY ON OUR SIDE

Ideally, we want those in the food industry responsible for the production of fruit, vegetables, and high-fiber grain products, as well as the producers and distributors of lower-fat meat and dairy products, to get more of their foods on food retailers' shelves. If you've ever tried to "healthy food shop" in smaller cities or towns and noticed the absence of fresh foods, or the absence of variety in "outside aisles," this is a food-industry and food-distribution problem. The first thing you can do is contact your local food retailers and ask them where they buy their produce, so you can contact the right channels to voice your concerns.

You may also notice that you can buy seven different kinds of brand-name cereals, but can't find a bag of natural oats or generic natural-grain cereals. Again, this is a food-industry problem, where brand-name, more-expensive, and less-nutritious products are often shelved because the profit margins are higher. In these cases, you can contact the food industry and make your demands known for more variety in products, particularly generic alternatives to brand names. Since the food industry is very concerned with what consumers want, they are more apt to respond to consumer demands. (See Appendix B for contact information.)

FOOD LABELS

Surveys continuously reveal that shoppers consider nutrition to be either very important or extremely important. They also reveal that consumers rely on packages and labels for nutrition information but, in most cases, find the ingredients list of certain products – especially processed and artificial food products – hard to decipher. In cases where food products are designed to mimic or substitute natural favorites like cheese, meat, and fish, consumers find assessing nutritional value difficult. We need labels that everyone can understand. In cases where it would be cumbersome to attach a label containing nutritional information to a food product (for example, a cinnamon bun baked in the store), perhaps the nutritional breakdown could be provided by the cashier at point-of-purchase.

So, who's responsible for our food labels? The state departments/ministries of health, agriculture, food, and rural affairs are chiefly responsible for developing nutritional labeling systems. If you're not happy with food labels, contacting these departments/ministries, as well as the product manufacturers, can help to bring about changes in the way nutritional information is presented.

MAKING SENSE OF LABELS

Nutritional information on food labels must make sense. In the United States, since 1993, food labels have been adhering to strict guidelines set out by the FDA and the USDA's Food Safety and Inspection Service (FSIS). All labels will list "Nutrition Facts on the side or back of the package." The "Percent Daily Values" column tells you how high or low that food is in various nutrients, such as fat, saturated fat, and cholesterol. A number of 5 or less is "low" – good news if the product shows <5 for fat, saturated fat, and cholesterol – bad news if the product is <5 for fiber. Serving sizes are also confusing. Foods that are similar are given the same *type* of serving size defined by the FDA. That means that five cereals that all weigh X grams per cup will share the same serving sizes.

Calories (how much energy) and calories from fat (how much fat) are also listed per serving of food. Total carbohydrate, dietary fiber, sugars, other carbohydrates (which means starches), total fat, saturated fat, cholesterol, sodium, potassium, and vitamin and minerals are given in Percent Daily Values, based on the 2,000-calorie diet recommended by the U.S. government. (In Canada, Recommended Nutrient Intake [RNI] is used for vitamins and minerals, while ingredients on labels are listed according to weight, with the "most" listed first.)

VITAMINS AND MINERALS FOR DAILY LIFE

- Vitamin A/beta carotene: Found in liver, fish oils, egg yolks, whole milk, butter; beta carotene: leafy greens, yellow and orange vegetables and fruits. Depleted by: coffee, alcohol, cortisone, mineral oil, fluorescent lights, liver "cleansing," excessive intake of iron, lack of protein.
- Vitamin B6: Found in meats, poultry, fish, nuts, liver, bananas, avocados, grapes, pears, egg yolk, whole grains, legumes.
- Vitamin B12: Found in meats, dairy products, eggs, liver, fish. Both B6 and B12 are depleted by: coffee, alcohol, tobacco, sugar, raw oysters, birth control pills.
- Vitamin C: Found in citrus fruits, broccoli, green pepper, strawberries, cabbage, tomato, cantaloupe, potatoes, leafy greens. Herbal sources: rosehips, yellow dock root, raspberry leaf, red clover, hops, nettles, pine needles, dandelion greens, alfalfa, echinacea, skullcap, parsley, cayenne, paprika. Depleted by: antibiotics, Aspirin and other pain relievers, coffee, stress, aging, smoking, baking soda, high fever.
- Vitamin D: Found in fortified milk, butter, leafy green vegetables, egg yolk, fish oils, butter, liver, skin exposure to sunlight, shrimp. Herbal sources: none; not found in plants. Depleted by: mineral oil used on the skin, frequent baths, sunscreens with SPF 8 or higher.
- Vitamin E: Found in nuts, seeds, whole grains, fish-liver oils, leafy greens, kale, cabbage, asparagus. Herbal sources: alfalfa, rosehips, nettles, Dang Gui, watercress, dandelions, seaweeds, wild seeds. Depleted by: mineral oil, sulphates.
- Vitamin K: Found in leafy greens, corn and soybean oils, liver, cereals, dairy products, meats, fruits, egg yolk, blackstrap molasses. Herbal sources: nettles, alfalfa, kelp, green tea. Depleted by: X-rays, radiation, air pollution, enemas, frozen foods, antibiotics, rancid fats, Aspirin.
- Thiamine (vitamin B1): Found in asparagus, cauliflower, cabbage, kale, spirulina, seaweeds, citrus. Herbal sources: peppermint,

burdock, sage, yellow dock, alfalfa, red clover, fenugreek, raspberry leaves, nettles, catnip, watercress, yarrow, briar rose buds, rosehips.

- Riboflavin (B2): Found in beans, greens, onions, seaweeds, spirulina, dairy products, mushrooms. Herbal sources: peppermint, alfalfa, parsley, echinacea, yellow dock, hops; dandelion, ginseng, dulse, kelp, fenugreek.
- Pyridoxine (B6): Found in baked potato with skin, broccoli, prunes, bananas, dried beans and lentils; all meats, poultry, fish.
- Folic acid (B factor): Found in liver, eggs, leafy greens, yeast, legumes, whole grains, nuts, fruits (bananas, orange juice, grapefruit juice), vegetables (broccoli, spinach, asparagus, Brussels sprouts). Herbal sources: nettles, alfalfa, parsley, sage, catnip, peppermint, plantain, comfrey leaves, chickweed.
- Niacin (B factor): Found in grains, meats, and nuts, and especially asparagus, spirulina, cabbage, bee pollen. Herbal sources: hops, raspberry leaf, red clover, slippery elm, echinacea, licorice, rosehips, nettles, alfalfa, parsley.
- Bioflavonoids: Found in citrus pulp and rind. Herbal sources: buckwheat greens, blue-green algae, elderberries, hawthorn fruits, rosehips, horsetail, shepherd's purse.
- Carotenes: Found in carrots, cabbage, winter squash, sweet potatoes, dark leafy greens, apricots, spirulina, seaweeds. Herbal sources: peppermint, yellow dock, uva ursi, parsley, alfalfa, raspberry leaves, nettles, dandelion greens, kelp, green onions, violet leaves, cayenne, paprika, lamb's quarters, sage peppermint, chickweed, horsetail, black cohosh, rosehips.
- Essential fatty acids (EFAs), including GLA, omega-6, and omega-3: Found in safflower oil, wheat germ oil. Herbal sources: all wild plants contain EFAs. Commercial sources: flaxseed oil, evening primrose, black currant, borage.
- Boron: Found in organic fruits, vegetables, nuts. Herbal sources: all organic weeds including chickweed, purslane, nettles, dandelion, yellow dock.
- Calcium: Found in milk and dairy products, leafy greens, broccoli, clams, oysters, almonds, walnuts, sunflower seeds, sesame seeds

(e.g., tahini), legumes, tofu; softened bones of canned fish (sardines mackerel, salmon), seaweed vegetables, whole grain, whey, shellfish. Herbal sources: valerian, kelp, nettles, horsetail, peppermint, sage, uva ursi, yellow dock, chickweed, red clover, oatstraw, parsley, black-currant leaf, raspberry leaf, plantain leaf/seed, borage, dandelion leaf, amaranth leaves, lamb's quarter. Depleted by: coffee, sugar, salt, alcohol, cortisone enemas, too much phosphorus.

- Chromium: Found in barley grass, bee pollen, prunes, nuts, mushrooms, liver, beets, whole wheat. Herbal sources: oatstraw, nettles, red clover, catnip, dulse, wild yam, yarrow, horsetail, black cohosh, licorice, echinacea, valerian, sarsaparilla. Depleted by: white sugar.

- Copper: Found in liver, shellfish, nuts, legumes, water, organically grown grains, leafy greens, seaweeds, bittersweet chocolate. Herbal sources: skullcap, sage, horsetail, chickweed.

- Iron (heme iron is easily absorbed by the body; non-heme iron is not as easily absorbed, so should be taken with vitamin C): Heme iron is found in liver, meat, and poultry; non-heme iron is found in dried fruit, seeds, almonds, cashews, enriched and whole grains, legumes, green leafy vegetables. Herbal sources: chickweed, kelp, burdock, catnip, horsetail, Althea root, milk thistle seed, uva ursi, dandelion leaf/root, yellow dock root, Dang Gui, black cohosh, echinacea, plantain leaves, sarsaparilla, nettles, peppermint, licorice, valerian, fenugreek. Depleted by: coffee, black tea, enemas, alcohol, Aspirin, carbonated drinks, lack of protein, too much dairy.

- Magnesium: Found in leafy greens, seaweeds, nuts, whole grains, yogurt, cheese, potatoes, corn, peas, squash. Herbal sources: oatstraw, licorice, kelp, nettle, dulse, burdock, chickweed, Althea root, horsetail, sage, raspberry leaf, red clover, valerian, yellow dock, dandelion, carrot tops, parsley, evening primrose. Depleted by: hot flashes, night sweats, crying jags, alcohol, chemical diuretics, enemas, antibiotics, excessive fat intake.

- Manganese: Found in any leaf or seed from a plant grown in healthy soil, seaweeds. Herbal sources: raspberry leaf, uva ursi, chickweed, milk thistle, yellow dock, ginseng, wild yam, hops, catnip, echinacea, horsetail, kelp, nettles, dandelion.

- Molybdenum: Found in organically raised dairy products, legumes, grains, leafy greens. Herbal sources: nettles, dandelion greens, sage, oatstraw, fenugreek, raspberry leaves, red clover, horsetail, chickweed, seaweeds.
- Nickel: Found in chocolate, nuts, dried beans, cereals. Herbal sources: alfalfa, red clover, oatstraw, fenugreek.
- Phosphorus: Found in whole grains, seeds, nuts. Herbal sources: peppermint, yellow dock, milk thistle, fennel, hops, chickweed, nettles, dandelion, parsley, dulse, red clover. Depleted by: antacids.
- Potassium: Found in celery, cabbage, peas, parsley, broccoli, peppers, carrots, potato skins, eggplant, whole grains, pears, citrus, seaweeds. Herbal sources: sage, catnip, hops, dulse, peppermint, skullcap, kelp, red clover, horsetail, nettles, borage, plantain. Depleted by: frequent hot flashes with sweating, night sweats, coffee, sugar, salt, alcohol, enemas, vomiting, diarrhea, chemical diuretics, dieting.
- Selenium: Found in dairy products, seaweeds, grains, garlic, liver, kidneys, fish, shellfish. Herbal sources: catnip, milk thistle, valerian, dulse, black cohosh, ginseng, uva ursi, hops, echinacea, kelp, raspberry leaf, rosebuds and rosehips, hawthorn berries, fenugreek, sarsaparilla, yellow dock.
- Silicon: Found in unrefined grains, root vegetables, spinach, leeks. Herbal sources: horsetail, dulse, echinacea, cornsilk, burdock, oatstraw, licorice, chickweed, uva ursi, sarsaparilla.
- Sulfur: Found in eggs, dairy products, cabbage family plants, onions, garlic, parsley, watercress. Herbal sources: nettles, sage, plantain horsetail.
- Zinc: Found in oysters, seafood meat, liver, eggs, whole grains, wheat germ, pumpkin seeds, spirulina. Herbal sources: skullcap, sage, wild yam, chickweed, echinacea, nettles, dulse, milk thistle, sarsaparilla. Depleted by: alcohol and air pollution.

THE SKINNY

If you're currently overweight or obese (as defined in Chapter 1), the key to losing weight is to begin a healthy diet. A healthy diet is about a balance of nutrients that incorporates all the food groups: carbohydrates, protein, and fat. Variety is the ticket. Whether it's a diet based on 55 per cent carbs/30 per cent protein/and 15 per cent fat or 40 per cent carbs/ 30 per cent protein/30 per cent fat – the ratio that allows greater flexibility – makes no difference unless you need to reverse dramatically signs of heart disease; in that case a very low-fat diet discussed in Chapter 4 is best. Be leery of fad diets that promise rapid weight loss (more than two pounds per week) and don't offer a balance of foods. Develop a critical eye about health claims made in various studies. Frequently the sponsors are revealed, which gives you a good indication about the agenda. Most important, keep in mind that dietary advice has remained constant over the years. The only thing that's changed is us: our lifestyle has become sedentary, and the food we ingest is largely fast food and convenience food. Meanwhile, as we all age, our metabolism changes, and we have to incorporate more activity into our lives if we want to eat the same number of calories we did even five years earlier. Our children's diets are reflecting the fast-food culture sold to them on television. There are no magic "eat all you want" diets (see Chapter 5); no magic pills (see Chapter 7). We need to wake up and realize the boring truth no one wants to hear. It's "grandma's rules": eat your vegetables; don't have cookies before dinner; no dessert tonight, you've had enough; go outside and play after dinner so your food digests better.

LINKS FROM SARAHEALTH.COM

For more information about disease prevention and wellness, visit me on-line at <www.sarahealth.com>, where you will find more than three hundred links – including these – related to your good health and wellness.

GENERAL HEALTH
- American Health Care Association: <www.ahca.org>
- The Canadian Medical Association: <www.cma.ca>
- American Medical Association: <www.ama-assn.org>
- Food and Drug Administration (FDA): regulations and information on drugs and other products. <www.fda.gov>
- National Institutes of Health (NIH): dedicated to providing the public with the latest information about different health issues and ongoing scientific research/special reports. <www.nih.gov>
- Center for Medical Consumers: <www.medicalconsumers.org>
- Intelihealth: <www.intelihealth.com>
- Health Information Highway: comprehensive health-care resource with discussion groups. <www.stayhealthy.com>
- Merck Manual: one of the most popular manuals used by doctors worldwide. Detailed information about thousands of conditions. <www.merck.com>
- Family Internet: information on diseases, conditions, treatments, prognoses, etc. With a health and diet file. <www.familyinternet.com>

DIABETES, BLOOD SUGAR, AND INSULIN INFORMATION

- American Diabetes Association: <www.diabetes.org>
- Canadian Diabetes Association: <www.diabetes.ca>
- American Association of Clinical Endocrinologists: <www.aace.com>
- National Institute of Diabetes and Digestive and Kidney Disease: <www.niddk.nih.gov/>
- Diabetes Resource Center: prevention, causes, signs and symptoms, treatment. <www.diabetesresource.com>
- About.com (Diabetes): <http://diabetes.about.com.health/diabetes/mbody.htm>
- Diabetes mall: targets both a general audience and medical professionals. Information about research, prevention, and education. With support group. <www.diabetesnet.com/index.php>
- Diabetes monitor: great source of patient information, research, statistics, and education. Registry of links. <www.diabetesmonitor.com>
- Olestra: information about this synthetic fat product now available in the U.S. <www.diabetesmonitor.com/olestra.htm>
- Recipe of the Day: features a new healthy recipe every day, Monday through Thursday. From the ADA. <www.diabetes.org/ada/rcptoday.html>
- Managing your Diabetes: official site of Eli Lilly & Co. Lots of great information about diabetes products. <http://lillydiabetes.com>
- Blindness and Diabetes Resource and Support: includes back issues of the "Voice of the Diabetic" from the National Federation of the Blind. <www.prevent-blindness.org>
- MedicAlert: site of the trademarked MedicAlert emblem. <www.medicalert.org>
- Diabetes Type 2, from the American Medical Association; symptoms, screening, diagnosis, complications, etc. <www.ama-assn.org/insight/spe_con/diabetes.htm>
- *Diabetic Gourmet Magazine*: free newsletter, daily tidbits, menus, and forum. <http://gourmetconnection.com/diabetic/>
- Health Net – Diabetes: treatment, patient education, advice. <www.healthnet.com>
- The Islet Foundation: dedicated to finding a cure for insulin-dependent diabetes. Interesting resources and information on the future of diabetes. <www.islet.org>

KIDNEY HEALTH
- The Kidney Foundation of Canada: <www.kidney.ca>

ON-LINE PHARMACIES
- <www.drugstore.com>
- <www.pharmweb.net>
- <www.cponline.gsm.com> (Clinical Pharmacology On-line)

DRUG DATABASES
- <www.rxlist.com>: free, searchable database of more than four thousand prescription and over-the-counter medications.

NATURAL/ALTERNATIVE MEDICATIONS AND THERAPIES
- <www.mothernature.com>: information on what natural remedies do and how to take them.

FINDING A DOCTOR
- Royal College of Physicians and Surgeons of Canada: <http://rcpsc.medical.org>
- American Medical Association: <www.ama-assn.org>

WHERE TO GO FOR
MORE INFORMATION

To find a dietician in your area, visit the Web site for the International Confederation of Dietetic Associations (ICDA), <www.internationaldietetics.org>. In Canada, you could also try <www.dieticians.ca>.

For inquiries about food products, labels, and health claims in Canada, contact:

Health Products and Food Branch Inspectorate Operational Centres

Atlantic
Suite 1625, 1505 Barrington St.
Halifax, Nova Scotia
B3J 3Y6
Tel: (902) 426-5350
Fax: (902) 426-6676
Note: Atlantic time

Manitoba and Saskatchewan
510 Lagimodière Blvd.
Winnipeg, Manitoba
R2J 3Y1
Tel: (204) 983-5453
Fax: (204) 984-2155
Note: Central time

Ontario
2301 Midland Ave.
Scarborough, Ontario
M1P 4R7
Tel: (416) 973-1466
Fax: (416) 973-1954
Note: Eastern time

Western
3155 Willingdon Green
Burnaby, British Columbia
V5G 4P2
Tel: (604) 666-3704
Fax: (604) 666-3149
Note: Pacific time

Québec
1001 ouest, rue St-Laurent
Longueil, Québec
J4K 1C7
Tel: (450) 646-1353, ext. 232
Fax: (450) 928-4455
Note: Eastern time

Diabetes/Hypoglycemia

*The Canadian Dietetic
Association*
480 University Ave., Suite 601
Toronto, Ontario
M5G 1V2
Tel: (416) 596-0857
Fax: (416) 596-0603

Alberta/N.W.T. Division
Suite 1010, Royal Bank Building
10117 Jasper Ave., N.W.
Edmonton, Alberta
T5J 1W8
Tel: (403) 423-1232
Toll-free: 1-800-563-0032
Fax: (403) 423-3322

Manitoba Division
102-310 Broadway Ave.
Winnipeg, Manitoba
R3C 0S6
Tel: (204) 925-3800
Toll-free: 1-800-782-0175
Fax: (204) 949-0266

*Canadian Diabetes Association:
National Office*
15 Toronto St., Suite 800
Toronto, Ontario
M5C 2E3
Tel: (416) 363-3373
Fax: (416) 363-3393

British Columbia/Yukon Division
1091 West 8th Ave.
Vancouver, British Columbia
V6H 2V3
Tel: (604) 732-1331
Toll-free: 1-800-665-6526
Fax: (604) 732-8444

New Brunswick Division
165 Regent St., Suite 3
Fredericton, New Brunswick
E3B 7B4
Tel: (506) 452-9009
Toll-free: 1-800-884-4232
Fax: (506) 455-4728

*Newfoundland/Labrador
    Division*
354 Water St., Suite 217
St. John's, Newfoundland
A1C 1C4
Tel: (709) 754-0953
Fax: (709) 754-0734

Prince Edward Island Division
P.O. Box 133
Charlottetown, Prince Edward
    Island
C1A 7K2
Tel: (902) 894-3005
Fax: (902) 368-1928

Saskatchewan Division
104-2301 Avenue C.N.
Saskatoon, Saskatchewan
S7L 5Z5
Tel: (306) 933-4446
Toll-free: 1-800-996-4446
Fax: (306) 244-2012

Food/Nutrition

National Institute of Nutrition
302-265 Carling Ave.
Ottawa, Ontario
K1S 2E1
Tel: (613) 235-3355
Fax: (613) 235-7032

Heart Health

*Heart and Stroke Foundation
    of Canada*
222 Queen St., Suite 1402
Ottawa, Ontario
K1P 5V9
Tel: (613) 569-4361
Fax: (613) 569-3278
Web site: <www.hsf.ca>

Nova Scotia Division
6080 Young St., Suite 101
Halifax, Nova Scotia
Tel: (902) 453-4232
Fax: (902) 453-4440

*Quebec CDA Affiliate:
Association Diabète Québec*
5635 Sherbrooke Ave. East
Montreal, Québec
H1N 1A2
Tel: (514) 259-3422
Fax: (514) 259-9286

Health Resource Centre
Tel: (416) 367-3313
Toll-free: 1-800-267-6817
Fax: (416) 367-2844
E-mail:heart@web.net
Web site: <www.web.net/ heart/>

BIBLIOGRAPHY

Addressing Obesity Early Birthkit: 5, Summer 1999. ISSN: 1075-4733.

"Affluent more prone to body image problems." (Nelliegrams) *Herizons*, 15 (4): 9(1), March 2002. ISSN: 0711-7485.

"Amy's story." *Girls' Life*, 8 (4): 50(5), February 2002. ISSN: 1078-3326.

Ashley, Mary Jane. Ferrence, Roberta. Room, Robin. Rankin, James. Single, Eric. "Moderate Drinking and Health: Report of an International Symposium." *CMAJ: Canadian Medical Association Journal*, 151(6):809-824, September 15, 1994.

Bacon, Jane G. Robinson, Beatrice "Bean" E. "Fat Phobia and the F-Scale-Measuring, Understanding and Changing Anti-Fat Attitudes." *Melpomene Journal*, 16 (1): 24-Spring 1997. ISSN: 1043-8734.

Beck, Kristin. "Baby Fat," *Moxie Magazine*: 14+, Summer 1999. ISSN: 1521-5873.

Blanco-Colio, Luis Miguel, B.S. Bustos, Carmen, Ph.D. Ortego, Monica, Ph.D. Hernandez-Presa, Miguel Angel, Ph.D. Cancelas, Pilar, Ph.D. Gomez-Gerique, Juan, M.D. Egido, Jesus, M.D. Valderrama, Monica, M.D. Alvarez-Sala, Luis Antonio, M.D. Millan, Jesus, M.D. "Conundrum of the 'French Paradox.'" *Circulation* Circulation (New York). 103(25):e132, June 26, 2001.

Branswell, Helen. "Women living in wealthy neighbourhoods less satisfied with own bodies: study." Canadian Press Newswire, F 11'02.

Broustet, J-P. "Wine and health." *Heart*. 81(5):459-460, May 1999.

Cameron, Debbie. "Sizing up the arguments." book reviewed: *Fat & Proud*. Cooper, Charlotte. *Trouble & Strife – the radical feminist magazine*: 5-11, Summer 1998.

Campos, Amparo Bonilla Carballo. Benlloch, Rosa Pastor. Martinez, Isabel. "Adolescence and Gender: Body Image and Eating Disorders." *Women's Health Collection*: 148+, No 06, 2001.

Center for Science in the Public Interest. "10 Super Foods You Should Eat!" *Nutrition Action Healthletter Online*. Posted to <http://www.cspinet.org/nah/10foods_good.html>. Retrieved 05/30/02.

——. "Cutting Cholesterol in Kalamazoo." *Nutrition Action Healthletter*, January/February 2002.

——. "FDA Fiddles While Americans Die." *Nutrition Action Healthletter*, April 2002.

——. "Rating the Diet Books." *Nutrition Action Healthletter*. May 2000. Posted to: <http://www.cspinet.org/nah/5_00/diet.htm>. Retrieved 05/30/02.

——. "Read My Lipids: How to Lower Your Risk of a Heart Attack." *Nutrition Action Healthletter*, October 2001. Posted to: <http://www.cspinet.org/nah/10_01/index.html>. Retrieved 05/30.

——. "Tax Junk Foods." *Nutrition Action Healthletter*, December 2000.

——. "Ten Tips for Staying Lean." *Nutrition Action Healthletter*, July 1999. Posted to: <http://www.cspinet.org/nah/7_99/ten_tips.htm>. Retrieved 05/30/02.

——. "Virtual Ingredients." *Nutrition Action Healthletter*, July/August 2001.

——. "What a Pizza Delivers." *Nutrition Action Healthletter*, June 2002. Posted to: <http://www.cspinet.org/nah/06_02/pizza_051702.pdf>. Retrieved 05/30/02.

——. "When in Rome: CSPI's Guide to Italian Food." *Nutrition Action Healthletter*, January/February 1994. Posted to: <http://www.cspinet.org/nah/ital.html>. Retrieved 05/30/02.

——. "Better than Butter?" *Nutrition Action Healthletter*, December 2001. Posted to: <http://www.cspinet.org/nah/12_01/index.html>. Retrieved 05/30/02.

——. "Label Watch: Ingredient Secrets." *Nutrition Action Healthletter*, July/August 2001. Posted to:

<http://www.cspinet.org/nah/07_01/ingredients.html>.
Retrieved 05/30/02.

Chalfen, Betsy. "Fats: The Good, the Bad, and the Fake."
Sojourner, 21 (7): 20, March 1996. ISSN: 0191-8699.

Cheng, T.O. "The Mediterranean diet revisited." *QJM*. 94(3):174-175,
March 2001. Held at Gerstein, U of Toronto.

Cheng, Tsung O. M.D. "Conundrum of the 'French Paradox.'"
Circulation|Circulation (New York). 103(25):e132, June 26, 2001.

Ducimetiere, Pierre, research director 1. Lang, Thierry, epidemiologist
1. Amouyel, Philippe, professor 2. Arveiler, Dominique,
epidemiologist 3. Ferrieres, Jean, epidemiologist 4. "Why
mortality from heart disease is low in France: Rates of coronary
events are similar in France and southern Europe." *BMJ*.
320(7229): 249, January 22, 2000.

Dunea, George. "Pinot Noir powders." *BMJ*. 319(7213):
861, September 25, 1999.

Eguia, Roberto. Bello, Alicia. "Anorexia and Bulimia: Early Prevention
and Detection." *Women's Health Collection*: 163+, No 06, 2001.

Friedman, Jeffrey M. "A War on Obesity, Not the Obese." *Science* 2003
299: 856-858. Volume 299, Number 5608.

Goldberg, Ira J., M.D. Mosca, Lori, M.D., Ph.D., M.P.H. Piano,
Mariann R., R.N., Ph.D. Fisher, Edward A., M.D., Ph.D. "Wine
and Your Heart: A Science Advisory for Healthcare Professionals
from the Nutrition Committee, Council on Epidemiology and
Prevention, and Council on Cardiovascular Nursing of the
American Heart Association." *Circulation*|Circulation (New York).
103(3):472-475, January 23, 2001.

Gopal, Kevin. "Weight-Loss Woes." *Pharmaceutical Executive*, 21 (11):
November 20, 2001. ISSN: 0279-6570.

Greenleaf, Christy. "Athletic body image: Exploratory interviews with
former competitive female athlete." *Women in Sport & Physical
Activity Journal*, 11 (1): 63(26), March 2002. ISSN: 1063-6161.

Gura, Trisha. "Having It All." *Science* 2003 299: 850. Volume 299,
Number 5608.

Haney, Daniel Q. "The Atkins diet's unlikely comeback."
Associated Press, February 16, 2003.

Hare, Suzanne. Drummond, Dianne. "Building body image: can parents
make a difference?" *Family Health* v. 17(4) Wint'01 pg 22-23.

Hoffmann, Carla. "Battle with body image – Eating disorders put many women's health at risk." *Sister Namibia*, 9 (3): 4-6, July 1997.

Hu, F.B., and Willett, W.C. "Optimal diets for prevention of coronary heart disease." *Journal of the American Medical Association*, November 27, 2002; 288(20):2569-78.

Kelner, Katrina and Laura Helmuth. "Obesity – What Is to be Done?" *Science* 2003 299: 845. Volume 299, Number 5608.

Ko, Marnie. "Blessed are the emaciated: even today's 'fleshy' celebrities are seriously underweight, and they're setting a terrible example." *Report Newsmagazine* v. 28(19) O 8'01, pp. 38-39.

Krane, Vikki. Waldron, Jennifer. Michalenok, Jennifer. Stiles-Shipley, Julie. "Body Image Concerns in Female Exercisers and Athletes: A Feminist Cultural Studies Perspective – Part 6" *Women in Sport & Physical Activity Journal*, 10 (1): 17, Spring 2001. ISSN: 1063-6161.

Kronberg, Sondra. "Nutrition & Eating Disorders – A Shared Journey" *Newsletter of the American Anorexia-Bulimia Association Inc*: 1-3, Fall 1997.

Lang, Maria. "My fat, My business! So all you fat-harassers out there, pay attention." *Radiance – The Magazine for Large Women*: 7, Summer 1996. ISSN: 0889-9495.

Langley, Susie. "Male body image obsession: the number of men with eating disorders and 'bigarexia' is rising." *Medical Post* v. 36(42) D 19'00, p. 34.

Law, Malcolm. Wald, Nicholas. "Attribution of time lag theory to explain French paradox." *BMJ.* 319(7216): 1073, October 16, 1999.

——. "Why heart disease mortality is low in France: the time lag explanation." *BMJ.* 318(7196): 1471-1476, May 29, 1999.

Losing Weight With Help – National Women's Health Report, 23 (1): February 6, 2001. ISSN: 0741-9147. Publisher: National Women's Health Resource Center.

Lutter, J. "Is Your Attitude Weighing You Down?" *Melpomene Journal*, Spring 1994. Mediamark Research Inc. Healthcare and Drug Products, Mediamark Research Inc., New York, N.Y., Spring 1994.

Lyons, Pat. "Losing Weight – An Ill-Fated New Year's Resolution." *Radiance – The Magazine for Large Women*, 15 (2): 8-9, Spring 1998. ISSN: 0889-9495.

——. "Fit AND Fat – An Idea Whose Time Has Come." *Melpomene Journal*, 15 (3): 4-8, Fall 1996. ISSN: 1043-8734.

Marx, Jean. "Cellular Warriors at the Battle of the Bulge." *Science* 2003, 299: 846-849. Volume 299, Number 5608.

Medcalf, Laura. "Beauty in the eye of the marketer: after a century of dictating an improbable body image, a few advertisers are leaving women be." *Marketing Magazine*, v. 102(38) O 13'97, pg 10.

Mickley, Diane. "New diet pill on the market." *Newsletter of the American Anorexia-Bulimia Association Inc*: 1-2, Fall 1996.

Miller, Mev. "Fat Politics – The Bottom Line is Women's Power." *Melpomene Journal*, 15 (3): 19, Autumn 1996. ISSN: 1043-8734.

"Most Girls Have Felt Unhappy with their Bodies." *Marketing to Women*, 14 (3): 12+, March 2001. ISSN: 1089-2958.

Nash, Madeleine J. "Cracking the Fat Riddle." *Time*, September 2, 2002: 46-55.

Nestle, Marion. *Food Politics: How the Food Industry Influences Nutrition and Health*. (2002, University of California Press, Berkeley).

Nichols, Mark. "Young and large: one of the pitfalls of obesity is that surplus weight, once acquired, is frustratingly difficult to shed." *Maclean's* (Toronto Edition), v. 113(20) My 15'00, pg 60.

Nutrition Action Healthletter, April 2002. Posted to: <http://www.cspinet.org/nah/04_02/index.html>. Retrieved 05/30/02.

O. Hill, James. Wyatt, Holly R. Reed, George W. Peters, John C. "Obesity and the Environment: Where Do We Go from Here?" *Science* 2003 299: 853-855. Volume 299, Number 5608.

Ontario Task Force on the Primary Prevention of Cancer. *Recommendations for the Primary Prevention of Cancer: Report of the Ontario Task Force on the Primary Prevention of Cancer*. [Toronto]: March 1995. Presented to the Ontario Ministry of Health.

"Overweight Women Make Less Money." *Marketing to Women*, 14 (1): January 12, 2001. ISSN: 1089-2958.

Parish, Lynn. "Mirror, Mirror." *Radiance – The Magazine for Large Women*: 32+, Fall 1994. ISSN: 0889-9495.

Paul, Noel C. "Whatever It Takes: More and more young men aim for the perfect body through pills, powders, and dietary supplements." *Christian Science Monitor*, 94 (125): 11+, May 22, 2002.

Peeke, Pamela. "Waistline Worries." National Women's Health Report, 23 (2): 8, April 2001. ISSN: 0741-9147.

Peters, Diane. "Don't hate me because I'm thin: get the skinny on what it's like to be slim in this weight-obsessed society." *Chatelaine* v. 73(6) Je'oo, pg 46.

"Physical Activity: A Treatment Option for Binge Eating Disorder?" [Part 2 of 3]. *Women in Sport & Physical Activity Journal*, 10 (2): 95(22), Fall 2001. ISSN: 1063-6161.

Pi-Sunyer, Xavier. "A Clinical View of the Obesity Problem." *Science* 2003 299: 859-860. Volume 299, Number 5608.

"Print Media: YM Magazine Swears Off Diet Stories." *Marketing to Women*, 15 (3): 8, March 2002. ISSN: 1089-2958.

Ravnskov, Uffe. "Why heart disease mortality is low in France: Miscoding may explain Japan's low mortality from coronary heart disease: Authors' hypothesis is wrong." *BMJ*. 319(7204): 255-256, July 24, 1999.

Rich, Lawrence Susan. "When Women Stop Hating Their Bodies." *Radiance – The Magazine for Large Women*: 20+, Fall 1995. ISSN: 0889-9495.

Rosenthal, M. Sara. *Stopping Cancer at the Source*. (2001, SarahealthPress, Toronto).

——. *The Canadian Type 2 Diabetes Sourcebook*. (2002, Wiley Canada, Toronto).

——. *Women and Passion*. (2000, Penguin Canada, Toronto).

——. *Women Managing Stress*. (2002, Penguin Canada, Toronto).

Rossiter, Kate. "Growing up girl." *Canadian Woman Studies* Wint/Spr'0120/21(4/1), pp. 89-91.

Sachiko T., St. Jeor, R.D., Ph.D. Howard, Barbara V., Ph.D. Prewitt, Elaine, R.D., Dr.P.H. Bovee, Vicki, R.D., M.S. Bazzarre, Terry, Ph.D. Eckel, Robert H., M.D. for the AHA Nutrition Committee. "Dietary Protein and Weight Reduction. A Statement for Healthc are Professionals from the Nutrition Committee of the Council on Nutrition, Physical Activity and Metabolism of the American Heart Association." *Circulation*. 2001; 104:1869-1874.

Samuels, Ellen. "Mixed Messages: Women and Dieting Culture: Inside a Commercial Weight Loss Group." Book reviewed: *Women and Dieting Culture: Inside a Commercial Weight Loss Group*. *Women's Review of Books*, 19 (3): 15(3), December 2001. ISSN: 0738-1433.

Schlosser, Eric. *Fast Food Nation: The Dark Side of the American Meal*. (2001, Houghton Mifflin, New York).

Sloan, A. Elizabeth, Ph.D. "Megamarkets, Nuances And Emerging Segments." *Natural Foods Merchandiser*: 16+, February 2002. ISSN: 0164-338X.

Stampfer, Meir. Rimm, Eric. "Why heart disease mortality is low in France: the time lag explanation: Commentary: Alcohol and other dietary factors may be important." *BMJ*. 318(7196): 1476-1477, May 29, 1999.

Stein, James H., M.D. Keevil, Jon G., M.D. Wiebe, Donald A., M.D. Aeschlimann, Susan, R.D.M.S., R.V.T. Folts, John D., Ph.D. "Purple Grape Juice Improves Endothelial Function and Reduces the Susceptibility of LDL Cholesterol to Oxidation in Patients With Coronary Artery Disease." *Circulation*\Circulation (New York). 100(10):1050-1055, September 7, 1999.

Stinson, Susan. "Nothing succeeds like excess." *Women's Review of Books*, XVIII (10-11): 16, July 2001. ISSN: 0738-1433.

Taylor, Catherine. "Women, Food, & Eating: An interview with two eating disorder specialists." *Radiance – The Magazine for Large Women*, 9 (1): 24+, Winter 1992. ISSN: 0889-9495.

"The 'New' Diet Pills: Buyer Beware." *Melpomene Journal*, 15 (3): 7, Fall 1996. ISSN: 1043-8734.

Torrance, Kelly. "Fat phobia: girls as young as five have started to count their calories." *Report Newsmagazine*, v. 28(5) Mr 5'01, pp. 64-66.

Toth, Emily. "Profiting from loss." Book reviewed: *Losing It – America's Obsession with Weight and the Industry that Feeds on It*. Fraser, Laura. *Women's Review of Books*, 15 (1): October 21, 1997. ISSN: 0738-1433.

Truelsen, Thomas, M.D. Gronbaek, Morten, M.D., Ph.D. Schnohr, Peter, M.D. Boysen, Gudrun, D.M.Sc. "Intake of Beer, Wine, and Spirits and Risk of Stroke: The Copenhagen City Heart Study." *Stroke*. 29(12): 2467-2472, December 1998.

Tunstall-Pedoe, Hugh. Kuulasmaa, Kari. Amouyel, Philippe. Arveiler, Dominique. Rajakangas, Anna-Maija. Pajak, Andrzej. "Myocardial Infarction and Coronary Deaths in the World Health Organization MONICA Project: Registration Procedures, Event Rates, and Case-Fatality Rates in 38 Populations From 21 Countries in Four Continents." *Circulation*\Circulation (New York). 90(1): 583-612, July 1994.

"Update – Prevalence of Overweight Among Children, Adolescents and Adults-United States, 1988-1994." *Morbidity and Mortality Weekly Report*, 46 (9): 199-202, March 7, 1997.

Urgo, Marisa. "Closing the Gap [Part 4 of 8]." *Closing the Gap*: 6+, 1998.

Vigilante, Kevin, M.D., M.P.H., and Flynn, Mary, Ph.D. *Low Fat Lies, High Fat Frauds*. (1999, Lifeline Press, Washington).

Visser, Marja. "Size Acceptance Outside The United States: The Netherlands." *Radiance – The Magazine for Large Women*, 13 (1): 32+, Winter 1996. ISSN: 0889-9495.

Wilson, G. Terence. "Understanding & Treating Obesity." *Newsletter of the American Anorexia-Bulimia Association Inc*: 1+, Fall 1998.

Wolf, Marina. "Fat Shoppers." *Radiance – The Magazine for Large Women*, 17 (3): 20, Summer 2000. ISSN: 0889-9495.

Wolfe, Charles D.A., M.D. Giroud, Maurice, M.D. Kolominsky-Rabas, Peter, M.D. Dundas, Ruth, M.Sc. Lemesle, Martine, M.D. Heuschmann, Peter, M.D. Rudd, Anthony, FRCP. (EROS) Collaboration. "Variations in Stroke Incidence and Survival in 3 Areas of Europe." *Stroke*, 31(9):2074-2079, September 2000.

"Women and Men Diet Differently." *Marketing to Women*, 13 (10): October 10, 2000. ISSN: 1089-2958.

"Women Dominate Dieting." *Marketing to Women*, 9 (1): January 6, 1996. ISSN: 1047-1677.

World Research Cancer Fund and the American Institute for Cancer Research. *Food, Nutrition and the Prevention of Cancer: A Global Perspective*. World Research Cancer Fund, 1997.

Yarnell, J.W.G. Evans, A.E. "The Mediterranean diet revisited – towards resolving the (French) paradox." *QJM*. 93(12): 783-785, December 2000.

INDEX